Cherisn tne Days

PLEASE RETURN TO:
COLEMAN WESLEYAN CHURCH LIBRARY
110 W. WEBSTER ST.
COLEMAN, MI 48618
(989) 465-6431

Compliments of...

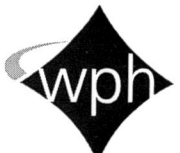 **wesleyan publishing house**

P.O. Box 50434
Indianapolis, IN 46250-0434

Call: 800.493.7539 • Fax: 800.788.3535
E-mail: wph@wesleyan.org • Online: www.wesleyan.org/wph

Please send copies of any review or mention.

Cherish the Days

INSPIRATION AND INSIGHT
FOR LONG-DISTANCE CAREGIVERS

MARTHA EVANS SPARKS

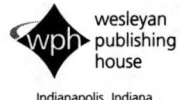

wesleyan
publishing
house

Indianapolis, Indiana

© 2004 by The Wesleyan Church. All rights reserved.
Published by Wesleyan Publishing House
Indianapolis, Indiana 46250
Printed in the United States of America
ISBN: 0-89827-272-6

Library of Congress Cataloging-in-Publication Data

Sparks, Martha Evans, 1927-
    Cherish the days : inspiration and insight for long-distance caregivers /
Martha Evans Sparks.
    p. cm.
    ISBN 0-89827-272-6 (pbk.)
    1. Caring–Religious aspects–Christianity. 2. Caregivers–Religious life. I. Title.
BV4647.S9S65 2004
259'.3--dc22
                                                                2004011637

No part of this publication may be reproduced, stored in a retrieval system,
or transmitted in any form or by any means–electronic, mechanical, photo-
copy, recording or any other–except for brief quotations in printed reviews,
without the prior written permission of the publisher.

All Scripture quotations, unless otherwise indicated, are taken from the HOLY
BIBLE, NEW INTERNATIONAL VERSION®. NIV®. Copyright 1973, 1978, 1984
by International Bible Society. Used by permission of Zondervan Publishing
House. All Rights reserved.

Scripture quotations marked (AMP) are taken from THE AMPLIFIED BIBLE,
Copyright © 1954, 1958, 1962, 1964, 1965, 1987 by The Lockman
Foundation. All rights reserved. Used by permission.

Scriptures marked (Jerusalem Bible) are taken from THE JERUSALEM BIBLE.
Copyright © 1966, 1967, 1968 by Darton, Longman & Todd Ltd and
Doubleday & Company, Inc.

Scriptures marked (The Message) are taken from THE MESSAGE. Copyright ©
1993, 1994, 1995, 1996, 2000, 2001, 2002. Used by permission of NavPress
Publishing Group.

Scripture quotations marked (NEB) are taken from THE HOLY BIBLE, THE
NEW ENGLISH BIBLE STANDARD VERSION, copyright © 1961, 1970 by Oxford
University Press and Cambridge University Press.

"Ten Warning Signs of Caregiver Stress" reproduced with the permission of
the Alzheimer's Association. Copyright 2004 Alzheimer's Association,
www.alz.org, 800.272.3900.

With love and appreciation to my parents,
Harry McDowell Evans and Mattie Harris Evans

Contents

Acknowledgments   9

Introduction   11

Chapter One   From a Thousand Miles Away:
               Dividing Caregiving Chores   13

Chapter Two   Hold On, Margaret, I'll Be Right There:
               Managing the Stress of Long-Distance Caregiving   27

Chapter Three Don't Disturb the Pickle Juice:
               Making Major Decisions   37

Chapter Four   You'd Better Come Right Away:
               Planning for Long-Distance Emergencies   49

Chapter Five   Polish Those Clubs Again, Dad:
               Identifying Creative Nursing Solutions   61

Chapter Six   Games People Play:
               Coping with Manipulative Family Members   73

Chapter Seven He Was My Father:
               Honoring Problem Parents   83

Chapter Eight I Forgive You, Mother:
               Repairing Broken Relationships   95

Chapter Nine   As Christ Loved Us:
               Caring for an Uncooperative Patient   105

Chapter Ten   Just One More Spin:
               Dealing with Unsafe Drivers   117

Chapter Eleven It's My House Now:
               Facing Legal Realities   127

Chapter Twelve Do You Think Mom's All Right?
               Selecting a Nursing Home   137

Chapter Thirteen   Your Dog Has Fleas:
                   Cherishing Family Memories   149

Afterword   157

Glossary of Caregiving Terms   161

Care Receiver's Information Packet   165

Ten Warning Signs of Caregiver Stress   169

Acknowledgments

To all of those who helped with this book I am grateful. To my friends who told me their long-distance caregiving stories: Susan Byars, Ernie Clarke, Rebecca Coyne, Susan Dummit, Jane Eakle, Janie Elliott, David Fleenor, Lynne Hollingsworth, Jerry Huffman, Esther Hurlburt, Kenton L. Kuehnle, Dr. George Lensing, Carol and Frank London, Mary Manassee, Nancy Menard, Anne Million, Cheri Perkins, Linda Pickerill, Sandi Prentis, Elizabeth Price, Judi Reid, Anne Marie Richard, Rudy and Nancy Rogers, Carol Rose, Linda Ruitenberg, Marlene Schlenther, Marie Smart, Dr. Christine Smith, Pat Taylor, Stanley and Evelyn Timblin, Annette Tornborg, Hazel Townsend, Lora Townsend, Whitlow Trumbull, Dr. Fred C. Van Tatenhove, Sarah White, Staci Wilder.

Also to Alan Beuscher; Steve Boven, Chief of Police, Wilmore, Kentucky; Steven Dawson, LCSW; Emily V. Evans; David Godfrey; Dr. Virginia Todd Holeman; Dr. Stuart Palmer; Eloise Griffith Penn; Marie Smart; Dr. Daniel Strait; and Lawrence W. Wilson, editorial director at Wesleyan Publishing House.

Introduction

"Long-distance caregiving is a mystery," says Eleanor. "You get on that airplane and wonder, *What will I find when I get there?*"

"I wish," she says, "there were someone in my parents' town I could call to look in on them—go to their house, look in the medicine cabinet, check the refrigerator, and look them over. I always have to wonder how they're doing; I never know for sure until I arrive." Eleanor lives in Tennessee, but she grew up in Idaho, where her parents still live. She is one of six siblings who now live in six states.

Eleanor's family is not unusual. In our highly mobile society, many people are separated from aging loved ones. Nearly seven million North Americans are long-distance caregivers. Many middle-aged children find themselves offering support, managing medical bills, and making long-term decisions for parents who live across town or across the country.

Caregiving is a growing industry. Advances in medicine continue to lengthen lives, but they do not always improve quality of life. The result is that almost one out of four households now cares for an aging loved one, three times as many as did so ten years ago. Seventy-five per cent of primary caregivers are women, the largest group being employed women in their forties and fifties. As the sheer number of caregivers increases, so does the realization that caregiving is a stressful, demanding task, emotionally and mentally exhausting.

This book contains the stories of some of these long-distance caregivers. If they are typical, then there is hope for us. The accounts of their loving determination to care for their aging parents across the miles is heartening—and sometimes heartrending. The task is incredibly demanding. Yet would they do it all again? Yes, indeed, they would. Why? "Because they are my parents" was the simple yet profound answer from all who share their stories in this book.

All of the narratives in this book are true. The names and most of the places have been changed to protect the privacy of the persons who gave so generously of their time and offered valuable insight into long-distance caregiving. This book would not have been possible without them.

If you are a long-distance caregiver, take courage. You are not alone. Read on to discover how others have struggled with and finally solved the problems of long-distance caregiving.

Chapter One

From a Thousand Miles Away
Dividing Caregiving Chores

Distance Dilemma   Coordinating care from a distance.

Caregiver Connection   Family unity bridges the distance between long-distance caregivers.

"All we wanted was to do the very best for Mom and Dad," said Susan Taylor Adams, "especially for Dad, after Mom died."

Doing the right thing for their aging parents turned out to be a challenge for Susan and her brothers, Joe and Alex Taylor. Their father announced early on that he would not move from his house in Columbia, South Carolina, where he had lived most of his life. Joe lived closest, a little over an hour away in Florence, South Carolina. Alex lived in Atlanta, a drive of some three-and-a-half hours. Eleven traffic-crammed hours of interstate highway lay between Susan's work in New York City and her childhood home.

Nobody planned for Ethel Taylor to die first. Albert Taylor, who was five years older than his bride, had assumed for more than fifty years that he would leave her a widow. Until then the two of them would live, as they had for decades, in the sprawling, comfortable, white, clapboard house where they had reared three children.

Neither had anyone believed that the vigorous couple would become physically handicapped; disability was something that happened to other people. But at the age of eighty-three, Albert began to complain of pain in his legs and feet. "At first we all hoped it would go away," says Susan, "but he was diagnosed with a circulatory ailment." Albert Taylor was soon dependent upon a wheelchair. He could no longer drive, a major problem for both him and his family. Ultimately, it was necessary to amputate one of his legs.

Ethel seemed healthier but was facing age-related problems of her own. Six months after the Taylors joyously celebrated their fiftieth wedding anniversary, Susan received a cryptic phone call.

"I was at the convention in Houston," Susan recalls. She had been a delegate to her church's national conference. "I was sitting in my hotel room when the phone rang. It was one of mom's neighbors."

"Did you know that your mother is not driving very well?" the caller asked.

"Um, no . . . I guess not," said Susan, her voice rising in concern.

It seems that Mrs. Taylor had left a church committee meeting and, instead of going down the driveway, had driven across the church lawn.

"I just thought you should know," the neighbor said, and hung up.

Susan paced the hotel room, filled with anxiety. *Did she think she was being kind by telling me?* Susan wondered, guilt and anger now mingling in her mind. *What am I supposed to do from a thousand miles away?*

The Distance Dilemma

Ever since our ancestors kissed their parents good-bye and rolled westward in covered wagons, Americans have gone where they've seen opportunity. When some of us accepted jobs on the other side of the continent from where our parents lived, it did not occur to us that Mom and Dad might someday need our care.

That realization comes suddenly. On the annual visit home, you notice how much Mom and Dad have changed since last year. *They look so old,* you think. Dad needs assistance with what were once routine tasks. The housekeeping is not up to Mom's usual standard. You spend an hour on the phone sorting out medical bills with the insurance company. You make one uncomfortable realization—*Mom and Dad need my help*—followed by another—*We live five hundred miles apart.* In that moment you enter one of the fastest-growing segments of our society, long-distance caregivers.

Whether it's across the country or just across town, distance creates a significant obstacle to caring for aging loved ones. More than seven million Americans are engaged in this worthy task, one laden with unique challenges.

Distance

Distance itself is the first problem for many caregivers. If your parents live in one place and your career has taken you to another, the miles become an obstacle to meeting your loved ones' needs. It doesn't matter whether the trip requires a transcontinental flight or merely fighting an hour of crosstown

15

traffic; you cannot drop by after work to see how the folks are doing today.

"My parents live in Idaho," says Eleanor, "and I live in Tennessee. Sometimes when I call them, they complain over little things, and I don't know whether to be concerned or not. At other times, they say, 'Oh, we're fine,' but I hear something in their voices that makes me wonder. I want to jump on the first airplane and go."

But she can't. Long-distance caregivers must find ways to keep tabs on Mom and Dad without being physically present all the time.

Immobility

In many cases, there is no way to close the distance gap. To the uninitiated, the solution appears simple. "Just have your parents move closer to you," they blithely offer. "Or maybe you could find a job in their town." Only two things are wrong with those suggestions: most parents won't consider moving, and most children cannot move their careers back home.

The Rollins family is typical. Earnest and Genevieve Rollins, now in their late eighties, lived in several New England states as Earnest's company transferred him from one assignment to another. Since retiring in the late 1970s, they have lived in the same house in Nashua, New Hampshire. To their three children, it is clear that the day-to-day management of the household has become too much, but the Rollinses will not consider moving. "We've moved enough," Earnest puts it bluntly. "It's time for us to stay put."

In fact, there is little alternative. "They can't move by themselves," says their son Jack, "and they won't let us help them." At this stage of life, the Rollins children agree that their parents

16

are incapable of managing the sale of their home and a cross-country move. They have waited too long.

In the meantime, the children have scattered, taking jobs where the best opportunities lay, as Americans have always done. None of the three can conveniently move back to New England to care for their aging parents.

Anxiety

Helplessness and frustration are the initial reactions to the realization that aging parents are in need of care. In shock and disbelief, we grapple with reality. As children, we took our parents for granted. Somehow, we thought they would always be able to care for themselves. But now we have reached the "wonder years."

- *I wonder how much longer they can live in this house.*
- *I wonder if they will be willing to move closer to us.*
- *I wonder if they can afford the cost of a retirement community.*
- *I wonder if they will have to live with us.*

All caregivers face these questions. For many, they are compounded by the distance that brings one more nagging thought: *I wonder if I'll be there when they need me.*

Family Stress

"The worst part was leaving the kids," says Susan Taylor Adams. Bona fide members of the *sandwich generation*, Susan Taylor Adams and her husband, Elliot, were in their late forties when Susan's father became physically incapacitated. About that same time, Susan's mother began to show symptoms of Alzheimer's disease. Susan and Elliot had three children living at home, and now aging parents were also in need of their attention. The Adams kids were good teenagers, and their parents trusted them; but the frequent trips to Columbia were hard on everyone. The children were left alone some, or they stayed with a neighbor.

"Even though our youngest could stay with friends while we were gone," Susan says, "she sometimes cried when we left." But what were the options? "Something was always going on with our parents," Susan recalls. She had little choice but to drive the eleven hours of interstate highway over and over again.

Miscommunication

The process of sharing information with and about aging parents can be like the children's game called Telephone. News is passed from one sibling to another until it becomes lost or distorted. And it's not a given that all members of an extended family will be happy to sit down together and plan for the care of aging loved ones. Sometimes a family meeting can be arranged, the problems discussed, duties divided up, and sometimes it can't. If a family has had trouble communicating in the past, the crisis of caregiving is not likely to improve the situation. Coordinating decisions among people living in different places is a challenge—even before family dynamics come into play.

The Beauty of Unity

"How good and pleasant it is when brothers live together in unity!" says Psalm 133:1. That scripture does not promise that everyone will concur on everything, but it does applaud those who agree to live and work together. The Lord must take quite seriously the matter of family unity because His word likens such accord to sacred anointing oil (Ps. 133:2). God gave to Moses the formula for compounding this holy oil, used in the consecration ceremony for priests. The Lord's instruction was to weigh definite amounts of myrrh, cinnamon, fragrant cane, and cassia, all very fragrant, and combine them in about a gallon of olive oil (see Exod. 30:22–25). The mixture was so hallowed that if it were used for anything other than the consecration of priests, the person who misused it was to be "cut off from his people" (Exod. 30:30–33). That oil and the unity that is likened to it are precious in God's sight.

Family unity not only pleases the Lord but also is beneficial to His people. Dew, the second figure of speech the psalmist uses to illustrate family unity, has long been a symbol of fruitfulness. "It is as if the dew of Hermon were falling on Mount Zion," says the psalmist (Ps. 133:3). Mount Hermon, a name that means *sacred mountain,* was near the northern boundary of ancient Israel. It is snow covered the year around, and its melting snows are the main source of the Jordan River. Some believe Mount Hermon to be the "high mountain" where Jesus' disciples saw Him transfigured (Matt. 17:1; Mark 9:2; Luke 9:28). Mount Zion refers to Jerusalem, so the psalmist is saying that unity is so beautiful and so important that it, figuratively speaking, refreshes the people of God. The unity of a family is no less precious in God's sight, and no less important for navigating the difficult road that is long-distance caregiving.

How is that unity achieved? Here are some practical steps for brothers and sisters to live together in harmony.

Focus on Those in Need

When aging parents need care, their needs must be primary. The first item for children to agree upon is that "It's our turn"— our turn to give, our turn to be responsible, our turn to sacrifice. Unity on that point is not always easy to achieve, for a number of reasons.

19

- *Rivalry.* Simmering family rivalries may exist, especially in blended families where "his," "hers," and "our" children may claim differing levels of responsibility for decision making.
- *Competing Needs.* Children in the sandwich generation often believe that the needs of their own children must take precedence over Mom and Dad's.
- *Confusion.* It may be difficult to determine the wishes of aging parents and how best to help them.
- *Selfishness.* Caregiving requires the sacrifice of time and, often, money. Some family members simply may be unwilling to part with either.

It may be necessary to confront the cause of division before unity can be achieved. Even during confrontations, the needs of the ill or aging loved one must be placed first.

Agree to Cooperate

Most often, the relationship between brothers and sisters will survive long after parents are gone. The issues discussed in family meetings will inevitably be emotional ones, and old tensions may come to the fore. But few of them—or none—are worth rupturing the family bond. Be flexible, be open-minded, and remember that the goal is always to care for the ailing loved ones, never to win an argument. Agree at the outset that you will work together and respect one another.

Discuss Finances Openly

Money is often the dominant issue in making caregiving decisions because nearly everything else is contingent upon it. That makes it essential for caregivers to be honest and cooperative in assessing family finances, particularly the finances of aging parents. Here are some of the questions that must be answered.

- What kind of health insurance do your parents have? Medicare does not cover all health care costs. Do they have a secondary insurance policy to cover at least part of what Medicare does not provide? Do they have insurance coverage for prescription drugs? Do they have long-term health insurance?
- Will your parents consider selling their home and moving to an apartment or condominium to reduce the cost and labor involved in maintaining their residence?
- Do your parents have enough income to pay the monthly fee in a retirement community?
- Are your parents able to afford the cost of remaining in their home, especially as they grow more dependent on assistance from others? Home care can cost up to three times as much as nursing home care.
- Would the sale of your parents' home yield enough for them to pay the entry fee at a retirement community offering the three levels of care: independent living, assisted living, and skilled nursing home care?
- If one of your siblings can provide adequate in-home care for the parents, will the others compensate her in some way for doing so? If one child takes a parent into her home, to what extent will your siblings help with expenses?

Amy, a medical professional who works with senior citizens, says, "It is no longer possible to get someone to help out of the goodness of their heart or in return for a small fee. Caring for old folks is hard work, and people want to be paid for it. If you have helpers in the home, be prepared to shell out big bucks." Money is a primary concern in caring for any dependent loved one. Caregivers must be prepared to discuss it early and to discuss it openly.

Be Tolerant

Every family must be prepared for the possibility that one or more members will not cooperate. Selfishness is usually at the root of the reasons family members are unwilling to share the burden of caring for aging parents; they do not wish to share their time or their money, and they leave the burden to others.

Danielle, who lives in Corvallis, Oregon, answered the telephone one afternoon to hear her brother, Jeff, asking, "Where are Mom and Dad this afternoon? They don't answer the phone. I called Dwight, and he didn't know either."

"My brothers live within ten minutes of our parents' home in Seattle," Danielle says, with some irritation. "Why do they call me, four hundred miles away, to ask something like that?" She answers her own question: "The unspoken message is that they don't care. They won't lift a finger to meet our parents' needs; they want me to do it all."

Yet Danielle wisely realizes that the insensitivity of her brothers is not worth losing their friendship. "I make the drive to Seattle whenever I can," she says. "Some things are worth fighting about, but that's not one of them."

Identify Helpers

It isn't only the children who can help out in the care of aging parents. Members of the extended family and even friends may be enlisted for support. You may not be as alone as you think. If a number of persons are each willing to assume a small responsibility, the load will not be quite so heavy for any one person. A neighbor may be willing to check the mail once a week for bills or other important items. A niece may be willing to provide transportation for doctor appointments. A friend from church might pick up Mom for trips to the grocery store. However, informal arrangements like these sometimes carry hidden dangers. (Read more on that in chapter 12.)

Develop a Plan

"We just knew," says Susan Taylor Adams. When it came time to divide up the tasks of caring for their father after Ethel Taylor's death, the Taylor children had an intuitive sense of which tasks each sibling was best suited for. They enlisted the help of others also. A housekeeper came in five days a week. An agency sent a helper each Saturday. Joe and his wife, Helen, came every Sunday to see how things were going and to take Joe's father to church and Sunday dinner, the high point of his week. Alex came about once a month for a long weekend, which he spent doing chores. Susan, the farthest away, came and stayed a week every two or three months. She brought financial records up to date, cleaned house, and in general tried to catch up. In between times, the three children made decisions by telephone.

Whether you "just know" or must have a family meeting to hash it out, it's vital to gain agreement on a workable plan for meeting the needs of the one receiving care.

Accept Risk

Life is risky, and so is caregiving. In order to offer care to a loved one, especially at some distance, you must be willing to accept that risk. Joe Taylor recalls that, much of the time, his father was left alone, a risky thing. But that uncertainty had to be balanced against the advantage of maintaining his father in his own home—Mr. Taylor's first priority. "The most important thing," Joe says, "is to do what the parent wants, and we did."

23

When well-meaning outsiders criticize your decisions, simply thank them for the advice and move on. As Joe points out, "Casual observers don't know the situation. You have to do what's best for your family." Gaining up-front agreement on major decisions makes it more likely that the family will stick together when questioned. Unity will be your ally when facing risk-filled situations.

Celebrate the Positives

Long-distance caregiving can turn into a positive experience. Clark and Marie, brother and sister, say they look forward to their caregiving visits to their mother as valued occasions to see each other. Their widowed mom lives in an assisted living community in the city where Clark and Marie grew up. Both have since moved away, and they sometimes plan to "meet at Mom's" when their spouses can join them. The occasions become family reunions.

"If Mom weren't living in our hometown, we probably wouldn't visit as much," says Clark. "But we make it a point to see old friends who still live there."

Hannah and Gary, another brother-and-sister team, have been pleasantly surprised by the blossoming relationship between them that has resulted from working together to care for their parents. "I've gained new respect for Gary," says Hannah. "I had always thought of him as my kid brother, not as a sensible man whose company I could really enjoy."

Perhaps the greatest reward for siblings who pull together is knowing that they have done their best to fulfill the Fifth Commandment, "Honor your father and your mother." As one long-distance caregiver put it, "One of these days my parents will die, and I don't want to be left wishing I had done more. I want to feel sure that I did everything I could have done, under the circumstances."

No Regret

"The next year was a nightmare," Susan Taylor Adams says candidly. After returning from the conference in Houston, she faced a series of trips to Columbia and dozens of conference calls with her brothers, which became their form of family meeting. The health of the elder Taylors continued to decline, and the first of a series of hard decisions had to be made. "We decided that Mom shouldn't drive anymore," Susan recalls. That resolution marked the beginning of eleven years of long-distance caregiving.

Ethel Taylor died of cancer three years after being diagnosed with dementia, leaving Albert disabled and alone. The Taylors, with careful money management, were able to keep their father in his own home for seven years after his wife's death. But with his condition weakening and his resources dwindling, the family was forced to make a difficult choice. When his house became his only remaining asset, Albert Taylor was placed in a nursing home paid for by Medicaid. He died less than a year later.

Reflecting on the experience, younger son Alex says, "I cannot imagine going through the eleven years we spent caring for our parents without unity among us. Bad as it was, we got through it because we worked together."

Helen Taylor, Joe's wife, saw that unity firsthand. "It was a learning process for me to listen to my husband and his siblings. They discussed issues and had differences, but they worked things out without anyone feeling pushed. It's over now, and they are still friends."

Older brother Joe agrees. "I have no guilt," he says calmly. "I am a realist and a businessman. In business, the worst thing you can do is not make a decision. Caring for aging parents is the same. We made the best decisions that we could, and I can live with that."

Sitting at the kitchen table, five years after her father's death, Susan Taylor Adams is a picture of serenity. The family conference calls are over—for this generation—there are no more hectic, anxiety-filled trips to Columbia. As she sits in the quiet of her suburban home, reflecting on the peaceful end of her father's life and the cooperation among her siblings that made it possible, Susan Taylor Adams echoes the hope of every long-distance caregiver. "We tried to do right by Dad," she says. "And I think we did."

Chapter Two

Hold On, Margaret, I'll Be Right There
Managing the Stress of Long-Distance Caregiving

Distance Dilemma   Preserving a home for aging parents.

Caregiver Connection   When family comes first, caregivers work
together.

amily always came first for the Hausers. Forty-eight-year-old
Rebecca remembers an idyllic childhood with her sister and two
brothers. Christmas gatherings at her grandparents' home were a
special treat. "They came to this country from Switzerland, and
they loved to have open house celebrations with family. There
might be thirty or forty of us for a sit-down dinner." The family
lived on a ranch in southern Arizona, and was somewhat isolated.
"But we were never bored," Rebecca insists. "The four of us played
together endlessly. We were like a modern Swiss family Robinson."

After the children were grown and gone, Rebecca's parents
sold the ranch and moved into the nearby city of Tucson. The

family began to scatter—Rebecca and her husband moved to Flagstaff and one brother to Los Angeles—but family ties were still close. They still enjoyed being together, and the Hauser home continued to be the focal point of extended family life.

"Then Dad got sick," Rebecca recalls. Armin Hauser had been the animated presence in the Hauser family. "My dad was actually the sociable one," Rebecca recalls. "Mom was a quiet person; she usually kept to herself." That made Mr. Hauser's battle with Parkinson's disease doubly challenging. As the disease progressed, Rebecca and her siblings were faced with two challenges: caring for their ailing father and keeping their family dynamics intact.

"I knew it would have been easier to put him in a nursing home," Rebecca recalls. "But Mom wouldn't hear of it."

"I'll not do it," Margaret Hauser insisted. "He'll lose his context for living—his home—his family."

"I knew she was right," Rebecca admits. "But how could we manage it? How could we both provide for Dad and keep the family life we'd always known?"

Caregiving and the Family

For Rebecca, her father's illness marked the beginning of two years of long-distance caregiving. Rebecca worked some sixty hours a week as an office manager, and she and her husband, Peter, drove five hours to Albuquerque once a month to visit their son, who was attending school there. Then, about once a month, she drove four hours to Tucson to spend a long weekend with her parents. "Those years are a blur in my memory," she remarks. "It was a very intense time."

That may be an understatement for Rebecca and the seven million other Americans who are long-distance caregivers. All caregivers are short on time and long on responsibilities. When distance is added to the situation, the problems are compounded. Here are a few of the difficulties Rebecca's family faced in trying to weather their family's home through the storm of long-distance care.

Stress

Seventy-five percent of primary caregivers are women, and the largest group of these is made up of employed women in their forties and fifties, like Rebecca and her sister. Margaret Hauser was the primary caregiver to her husband, but the daughters played strong supporting roles. Members of the sandwich generation—caught between caring for both aging parents and at-home teenagers—they were overloaded with responsibilities. Having only the usual twenty-four hours in each day, the girls became short on time for cultivating their marriages, attending children's ballgames, or doing things for themselves—including sleeping.

The inevitable result of that hectic schedule is stress—stress on marriages, on business relationships, and on children. Volunteer work, entertaining, and even quiet evenings alone become a distant memory.

Relational Tension

And there were stresses within the family as well. "Caregiving for our parents was like walking through a minefield," says Rebecca. "We did not want to usurp our mother's decision making, so sometimes we got into a kind of dance routine where we tiptoed around problems." Eventually those tensions reached a crisis point. "We were trying to keep Mom happy, but there were times when decisions absolutely had to be made. It got complicated at times."

29

Unequal Load

Rebecca's sister and one brother lived only minutes from their parents' home in Tucson, so the heaviest caregiving load fell upon them. While the siblings were able to hire nursing assistants to provide morning care for their father, either the brother or sister living nearby stopped by each night to get their father into bed.

"I began to see my job as caring for my sister," says Rebecca, who often lent a listening ear at one end of a long-distance phone call. "I also did Mom's shopping during my monthly visits, then spent the rest of the weekend cooking." Rebecca's visits were a help, but didn't nearly equalize the caregiving load among the siblings.

An unequal division of labor is typical for long-distance caregiving families. That inequality, however unavoidable, can become a source of tension among family members.

Helplessness

Like Rebecca's father, Elaine's dad developed Parkinson's disease. The effects of the disease have been particularly cruel in her father's case. A retired teacher, his daughter describes him as "an incredibly articulate man." Now he cannot speak. He was an excellent craftsman and woodworker. Now the disease has robbed him of his fine motor skills. Elaine is anguished over her father's disability. "It's been so painful to watch this disease ravage his body. I prayed for two or three years that the Lord would take him," she admits. But that hasn't happened. He lives on in increasing disability.

Holly, who lives in North Carolina, knows the feeling. "The hardest thing," she says, "is seeing my mother lying there helpless but with full command of her mental faculties. It's pitiful."

Holly's mother lives in a rehabilitation facility, but Holly still provides a good deal of care, even though she lives more than an hour away. "When I change her diaper, she cries and says, 'I didn't want you to ever have to do this.'" Like many long-distance caregivers, Holly, too, has prayed for the end. "I sometimes pray, *O God, let this be over*. But then I feel guilty for thinking that way."

Helplessness followed by frustration and guilt is a progression of emotions well known to long-distance caregivers.

The Source of Hope

The Apostle Paul said, "Do not be anxious about anything, but in everything, by prayer and petition, with thanksgiving, present your requests to God" (Phil. 4:6).

"That sounds good," says the harassed caregiver. "But I'm still short of sleep and have a lot of tough decisions to work through. I need more than nice-sounding words."

Yet the next verse in Paul's letter puts our hope on a more active footing by using a military term. Philippians 4:7 promises that if you do present your requests to God with thanksgiving, "The peace of God, which transcends all understanding, will guard your hearts and your minds in Christ Jesus." The Greek word translated *guard* is a military term that means to post a sentinel or to protect with a garrison of soldiers.

Picture the peace of God pulling guard duty over your heart, keeping watch over your feelings and emotions. If we have offered sincere prayer to God, then we can claim the promise that His peace will be on guard against anxiety, frustration, anger, bitterness, depression—all of the emotions that threaten to overwhelm us. And realize that this peace actively guards our minds as well. Under the command of God's guardian peace, our mind's knowledge and reasoning powers become strong,

31

disciplined soldiers, ready to help us deal with the isolation and stress that so often besiege caregivers. God, invited into our lives through the practice of daily prayer, can keep us from hitting the brick wall at the end of the dead-end alley of our own strength.

Here are some practical ways that God's peace works in our lives.

Develop Devotional Disciplines

With a mixture of tears and laughter, Rebecca recounts how she, her husband, Peter, and their siblings survived two years of frequent hospitalizations of her father, midnight telephone calls from the hospital, long drives at odd hours, and the grind of fulltime work and weekend caregiving. "In that chaos, the Lord supported me," she says. "I learned the absolute necessity of devotional life. I needed forty-five minutes or an hour in God's Word every day. That discipline paid the rent."

Caregivers are habitually short of time, but time spent with God is not a luxury; it is a necessity. When the demands of work, family life, and caregiving begin to crowd good activities out of the schedule, resist the urge to sacrifice the discipline of devotional life. Time with God provides the refreshment that will keep you going.

Seek Christian Community

Rebecca also drew strength from close association with God's children. "I have two very close women friends; one in particular is a rock for me," she says. This woman was a comrade ready to listen on the telephone, share a prayer, and assist with decision making.

Then there was the early morning prayer group. Every Thursday at 6:00 a.m., Rebecca met with a group of women for prayer. "It's a covenant group," she explains. "We've been through the wars with our kids and with our parents. I would trust any of them with my life." The intimacy of that close-knit group provided invaluable support. "When you meet at 6:00 in the morning, just one step out of your pajamas, you get to know people really well," Rebecca says laughingly. "I really benefited from those relationships."

Embrace the Experience

"I know what it means to be ground down to nothing," Rebecca says. "I've been there." But that doesn't mean the veteran caregiver offers easy answers or cheap advice to those who suffer. "I tell people that their hope is in Jesus," she says candidly. "The Lord gives us these trials as a refiner's fire. It's hard to appreciate that in the midst of the flames, but I know that I am a richer, deeper person for what I've been through. It was my privilege to suffer."

Easy advice? Hardly. But Rebecca knows, just as James did centuries ago, that God often works best in our lives when we suffer trials (see James 1:2–5). When we can be thankful to God, even in the worst circumstances, we will grow by what we suffer.

Pray

"My advice to caregivers is pretty simple," says Rebecca. "Pray. Give the entire situation to the Lord; that's where our hope lies." Sometimes those prayers are hard to come by. Fatigue and frustration bring doubts to the caregiver's mind. Exhaustion makes it difficult, sometimes impossible, to concentrate on conversation with God. When that happens, call others and enlist their prayer support. God is faithful; He will bring the peace that He promised in response to your trusting call.

Hold On, I'll Be Right There

After two years of concerted effort, the Hauser family had succeeded in preserving their family life. Armin, increasingly debilitated from his disease, was cared for at home. Margaret, supported by her children and some outside help, was able to manage her husband's care. The family was stretched thin, but it was holding together. Then the unthinkable happened: Margaret Hauser died.

"She'd had surgery," Rebecca remembers, "and something happened during her recovery. By the time we arrived, it was pretty clear this was the end." With several family members present, Rebecca anointed her mother and prayed. "Then we let her go," Rebecca says calmly. Assured of her salvation, it was Rebecca's privilege to usher their beloved mother into the presence of God.

But what about their father? What about the family's dream of preserving his home life? How would they manage his care with their mother gone?

After the memorial service for Margaret, Rebecca and her three siblings brought their father, in his wheelchair, to his beloved wife's gravesite. His Parkinson's disease had advanced so far that Armin could neither walk nor speak. The children silently wondered how their father would react, if at all, to the event. The ailing man looked at his children, lined up around the grave with their spouses and his grandchildren. He examined them carefully, then closed his eyes. All of his children were sure he was inwardly repeating the words he had said for years during any household emergency, *Hold on, Margaret, I'll be right there.*

"Right then, he set his mind on dying," Rebecca says emphatically. "My father willed himself to be alive for my mother. If her job was to take care of him, then his job was to stay alive for her. Now he was free to go."

Four days later, Armin Hauser died.

"After Mom and Dad died within a week of each other," says Rebecca, "friends asked us how we were going to cope with it. But we all knew it was a gift from the Lord." Their mother had been spared a long illness and the torture of a slow death. Her father had finally been freed from the prison of Parkinson's disease. Through it all, they had been wonderfully, beautifully cared for, surrounded by the attention of a devoted family. Now they are united again, in heaven. "It was a bittersweet ending," Rebecca admits. "Those years were difficult, but I look at our sacrifice as a monument to our parents."

And with the Hausers, family always came first.

Chapter Three

Don't Disturb the Pickle Juice
Making Major Decisions

Distance Dilemma	Knowing when to make lifestyle changes for care receivers.
Caregiver Connection	Respecting care receivers' wishes leads to peace.

"As soon as my mother began to show symptoms of Alzheimer's disease, my father announced that they were not going to move. He said he could take care of her all by himself, right there in her own home." Anne Middleton's father was raised on self-reliance. When he saw a need, he met it. "And he was quite capable of managing this circumstance," Anne adds. "At least in the beginning."

Anne's parents, George and Beulah Kohler, had lived all of their adult lives in Clayton, Oklahoma, population less than one thousand, in the same house where Anne and her sister, Jean, grew up. They knew everybody in town. Anne and Jean lived about an equal distance from Clayton, but in different directions. It took about four hours for Anne to drive up from Dallas; Jean had a similar drive from her home in Oklahoma City.

As Beulah's dementia deepened, George shouldered added responsibilities. He began doing all the driving and shopping, then the cooking, and finally even the laundry and household cleaning. He was a vigorous, determined man, and he handled the added load without much problem. For several years Anne and Jean watched with increasing concern as the inevitable signs of aging crept over George.

"I worked on getting them to move for five years," "Anne reports. "We saw a crisis looming and we tried to prevent it. Dad looked at it differently." The sisters merely wanted for their parents to be surrounded by people who could help them. George Kohler was intent on maintaining his home and his independence. Reluctantly, the daughters came to see that their vision of their father's life was not necessarily what he wanted—or what was best. The girls visited upon occasion and kept in touch by telephone. George was always upbeat. "Everything is fine," he would say, although sometimes his daughters wondered.

Then it happened. One day Anne received a call from a panicky George Kohler. "Anne, I can't find mother. She's wandered out of the house."

To Move or Not to Move

Anne and Jean faced a dilemma encountered by many long-distance caregivers: when, if ever, do you compel loved ones to make a major lifestyle change in order to facilitate their care? How do you know when it's time to take control of the situation? Should you ever pressure loved ones to move? When is it right to place Mom in a nursing home without her consent? These questions are bursting with difficult issues. Here are some of the problems that can encumber the thorny decisions surrounding long-distance caregiving.

Caregiver Motivations

Long-distance caregivers, eager to end the commute between their homes and that of their care receivers, may allow their judgment to be clouded by the miles. Within a week of her father's death, Anita was urging her mother, Sophia, to sell the family home and move into a retirement community. Anita lives in Seattle. Her parents lived in Greensboro, North Carolina. Without recognizing the transparency of her words, Anita flatly told a friend, "I'm anxious to get Mom settled somewhere close so I won't have to make trips across the country to check on her."

Long-distance caregivers especially need to ensure that their motives are selfless, giving priority to the welfare of the care receiver. The caregiver's financial, physical, and emotional resources are factors, to be sure. It can be tricky to decide whether a decision is being made for the caregiver's convenience at the expense of the loved one's comfort. Rachel, whose parents live two hours away from her, says, "This is not just about our peace of mind. It's about tearing the fabric of another person's life. As they get older, our parents are no less persons than they ever were."

Caregivers must be certain of their motives before insisting on a change.

Lack of Sensitivity

"Your parents are unique people," says Rachel, who presents seminars for senior citizens and their adult children. "They are not simply older versions of you."

Caregivers sometimes assume that they know what their care receivers desire or what is best for them. They don't, always. "Try to look at things from the care receiver's viewpoint," suggests Doris, who struggled with a decision about when or whether to compel her parents to move into assisted living. "Suppose someone walked up to you and said, 'I don't think you're managing your life very well. You need to move out of your home.' How would that make you feel?"

It is true that aging parents sometimes revert to acting like children, but they should not be treated as if they were not equals at the table. They should have a voice in any decision concerning them. "I had to be flexible," says Doris, "and willing to negotiate and compromise with my parents as I would with any business associate."

Overprotection

It may be difficult to distinguish the difference between harmful behaviors by aging parents and activities that are merely eccentric. Ellen, whose father had moved to Florida, learned not to sweat the small stuff. Once when she went for a visit, she found six quarts of pickle juice in the refrigerator. "I left it alone," Ellen relates, "because I was sure Dad must have had some reason for keeping it." Sure enough, he did. "He said it made an inexpensive salad dressing. Who knew?"

Yet some eccentric behaviors are really symptoms of the care receiver's inability to cope with independent living. If some adult children live in denial of the alarming changes in their parents' mental capacity, some others overreact, seeing danger in every unusual but otherwise harmless situation. It can be difficult to decide whether a situation poses a serious risk and warrants taking the initiative in changing aging parents' lifestyle.

Unintended Consequences

Judith made frequent two-hour drives to her parents' home for several months during her father's illness. After he died, she believed she had the authority to confront her mother with some needed changes. "It backfired," Judith confesses. "Mom attempted suicide rather than move out of her house into an apartment." A safe move to more manageable living quarters was finally accomplished after psychiatric counseling, but the lesson wasn't lost on Judith. "It's very hard to predict the consequences of a forced change," she warns.

Ignorance

"My brother's wife always wants to change things," says Ralph. His mother had a shabby overstuffed armchair in her living room, and everybody agreed that it looked appalling. Ralph's sister-in-law decided to amend the situation by hauling off the old chair and replacing it with a new one. "But she didn't ask if Mom wanted a new chair," Ralph continues. "Mom was so shocked that she didn't say anything at first. Then she got angry. To this day my sister-in-law can't understand why Mom doesn't like her very much."

As it happens, the tattered old chair was the first piece of furniture Ralph's parents bought after they married. Besides the sentimental value, the fluffy cushions felt "just right" to Mom's arthritic back. The well-meaning daughter-in-law might have known those things if she had asked.

Caregivers—or would-be helpers—sometimes jump to wrong conclusions about the living situations of their care receivers. Those who don't know what they don't know often make mistakes.

41

Knowing when to press for change in a care receiver's lifestyle is seldom simple. Most caregiving situations are clouded by difficult emotions, which may be compounded by distance. So how can we know when to move and when not to?

Calm amid the Storm

"Peace to you," John closes his third letter (3 John 14). "Peace I leave with you; my peace I give you," said Jesus to the disciples at the Last Supper (John 14:27). The author of the letter to the Hebrews ascribes to "the God of peace" power so strong it "brought back from the dead our Lord Jesus." The writer goes on to say that this same power is available to equip us for doing God's will (Heb. 13:20, 21). In fact, the tenor of the entire Bible is that God's people should allow God to maintain His peace within them, no matter how tempestuous the events on the surface of their lives may be.

The final test in Christian decision making is peace. Regarding a difficult decision, we often ask one another, "Do you have God's peace about it?" After you have assembled the information, learned as best you can, consulted with those genuinely concerned with the matter, considered possible consequences, consulted Scripture, prayed with an open heart, and listened for the voice of God, the one thing that remains is to gain a sense of God's peace. That inner confidence is the last prerequisite for taking action. Without it, no plan will likely succeed. With it, you will be able to better cope with the difficulties, even heartaches, that so often follow caregiving decisions.

That peace will ultimately come to your heart from the heart of God. As you seek His peace, these simple steps may assist you in untangling the thorny questions that surround the decision to make a major lifestyle change for your care receiver.

Investigate Options

When it becomes apparent to you that aging loved ones need to make some fundamental change in living arrangements, the first thing caregivers should do is investigate alternative living arrangements. While it is important to include care receivers in the decision making process, it is best to develop a plan in advance that can be presented to the care receiver for input and approval. Arrange a family meeting or conference call that includes everyone who has a stake in the decision. Be straightforward in listing the problems you see. Work together to evaluate alternatives, including investigating assisted living facilities, nursing homes, retirement communities, adult day care facilities, or other care facilities. Develop a plan tailored just for your care receiver.

Preplan a Compromise

Compromise is a fact of life in caregiving. It's quite likely that your first plan will not work out entirely. The care receiver may balk at the plan. Arrangements may have to be postponed because of illness. Windows of opportunity sometimes close. It's essential to have plan B and possibly even a Plan C in mind.

Alberta, who made frequent hour-and-a-half drives from her home in Baltimore to her parents' home in Lancaster, Pennsylvania, says, "After my father's death, I wanted to move Mom into an apartment near me, but she wouldn't leave her friends. We compromised, and she moved into an apartment in Lancaster. I still had a long drive, but I did not have to go as often."

Investigate second and third options for your care receiver's living arrangements. One of them will likely be acceptable for all concerned.

Count Care Receivers In

It cannot be emphasized too strongly that if mentally able, care receivers must be included in discussions about changes in living arrangements. What could be more arrogant than to make life decisions for other people behind their backs? After doing some preliminary planning, sit down with your care receivers and share your thinking with them honestly, supporting your reasons for believing a move is necessary. It is extremely important that care receivers make the final decision to alter their lifestyle, if they are competent to do so. Remember Jesus' Golden Rule: "Do to others as you would have them do to you" (Luke 6:31).

Plan an Approach

After arriving at your carefully made plan, decide on the most effective way to present it to your care receiver. Tact and grace will be your allies. "We didn't just announce 'This is the way it's going to be,' says Agnes, who struggled through years of long-distance care before being able to convince her parents to move into more manageable housing. "We went to Mom and Dad with a plan; but we were prepared to change it, and we told them so." In fact, the plan did change several times before finally being implemented. After many long discussions, Agnes's mother finally said, "We'll do whatever you think is best." Agnes's tactful, nonthreatening approach laid the groundwork for that moment of openness.

Prove Your Case

Connie's father insisted he could manage alone. He did not recognize that he was able to care for his infirm wife only because Connie made frequent four-hour trips between her home in Albuquerque and his place in Roswell, New Mexico. A social worker advised Connie, "Back off a little. Let him do more of the work."

"It was hard to do," Connie admits, "but I went home early from one trip and let him bear the burden." The lesson was quickly learned. "I got a call the next day," Connie says. "Dad was ready to admit that Mom should go into assisted living."

Lovingly but honestly, find ways to show your care receivers how dependent they are. Remember that this lesson is humbling to learn. Be gentle, but allow the truth to be seen.

Involve a Mentally Impaired Care Receiver

In cases where a care receiver is mentally impaired, a good faith effort should be made to explain the plan to him or her. The discussion should be held in terms the care receiver can understand, and there must be no hint of condescension or belittling. A longer, more detailed discussion can follow when caregivers meet with doctors, lawyers, bank personnel, real estate professionals, or other persons to finalize plans.

Accept What Cannot Be Changed

Sometimes care receivers simply will not agree to move. It may be necessary to continue making long or inconvenient trips until they realize that another lifestyle will make it easier for both the caregiver and themselves.

When care receivers insist on maintaining their independence in spite of some risks, it is important not to fall victim to guilt. Some things about the care receiver's life may simply look strange, like the pickle juice Ellen found in her father's refrigerator. Some others may be dangerous. But there are times when an adult's way of life cannot be changed without riding roughshod over the will and rights of a person whose only crime is having grown old.

Laurie's mother, who lived alone, fell and lay on the floor of her home for two days before being discovered. "I felt terrible about it," says Laurie, "like I had failed her." Laurie should not have blamed herself. Her mother's repeated refusal to move into an assisted living facility—in spite of Laurie's best efforts to persuade her to do so—created a risky situation that was beyond Laurie's power to change.

Most persons with normal mental capacity will be sensible enough to comply with lifestyle changes that will increase their comfort and security. Lovingly but honestly find ways to show your care receivers how dependent they are. Above all, do not patronize. No one will be inclined to agree with your suggestions, much less your instructions, if they are seen as condescending.

The Place of Peace

Anne Middleton hung up the phone and raced to her parents' home in Clayton, Oklahoma. To Anne's great relief, her mother had been found about a block from home, but the incident had forced a crisis. "That day Jean and I began making alternate weekend trips to visit our parents," Anne recalls. "Mom's wandering meant Dad was on call twenty-four hours a day, but he still wouldn't agree to assisted living."

The weekend trips continued for several years, during which Anne and Jean tried to persuade their father to move into an assisted living facility near Jean's home in Oklahoma City. "Goodness knows it would have been easier on us if they moved sooner," Anne laments. "But it had to be his decision.

Dad had to progress at his own speed toward the decision to leave their home."

Then came another call.

"Anne, I'm sorry to bother you," George Kohler began, "but your Mom has fallen and hurt herself. I may need a little help."

Anne made the drive to Clayton and stayed for a week, leaving only when George insisted that she return home. But the very next day, she received another call, this one from a friend of her father's at church. "Your dad is overwhelmed," the caller said. "I think he's really at the end of his rope. Can you come back?"

Anne drove to Clayton immediately, where she found her father wearily sitting in the kitchen. "I can't do this anymore," he finally admitted, his head hung low. "I think we need to get your mother some help." After several long discussions with Anne and Jean, who had also returned to Clayton, George finally agreed to move.

"It was hard to move them," Anne recalls. "But it was his decision. He agreed to move into the same assisted living facility we had selected years before." The years of commuting were difficult, but Anne has no regrets. "I'm proud of my Dad," she says with a smile. "He was one of those stubborn German Lutherans, strong people who can stand just about anything. But when he couldn't take it anymore, he made his own choice to move."

And the move came just in time. Two months later, as the Kohlers were just settling into their new apartment, George died after being hospitalized for only three days. "I'm just thankful I got to be there through it all," says Anne. "With tears and hugs, it was a cleansing time for us." Adding to the sisters' relief was the knowledge that they had treated their father with dignity, respecting his ability to make decisions for their mother. "When he breathed his last, we experienced a peace—a peace that descended. It was a very sacred time."

As John has said to us all, "Peace to you" (3 John 14).

Chapter Four

You'd Better Come Right Away
Planning for Long-Distance Emergencies

Distance Dilemma	Having a ready response to medical emergencies.
Caregiver Connection	Prior planning eases the burden of long-distance care.

"Strokes happen fast," says Greg Marler. "I was totally unprepared for what happened to Dad." Greg received the phone call every long-distance caregiver dreads one day at his Fort Collins, Colorado, home.

"It's your father," Cleo Marler said, her voice faltering. "You'd better come down right away."

Gene and Cleo Marler lived in Pueblo, about three hours south of Fort Collins. Greg jumped into his car and drove down, having no idea what to expect when he arrived. His father survived the stroke but was unable to return home from the hospital. He was placed in a nursing home, leaving Cleo alone at home.

"That was the beginning of my weekend commuting," says Greg. The routine was predictable. Every other Friday, Greg left work a little early, arriving in Pueblo near suppertime. After a visit with his mother, he headed to the nursing home to check on his dad. On Saturday mornings, Greg made sure the bills had been paid and made small repairs on the house. He returned home to Fort Collins on Saturday afternoon or Sunday morning.

This went on for six years.

It would have been easier on Greg to move his parents north, but he resisted the change as much as they did. "Dad built that house after the war," Greg explains, meaning World War II. Gene and Cleo were proud members of what has been called the greatest generation. "The place was full of memories for all of us."

But the years of commuting took their toll on everyone. Cleo Marler's health was beginning to fail, Greg was tiring of the biweekly drive, and his wife, Carla, was feeling the strain.

"She shouldn't be left totally alone, Greg. I think it's time to make some changes."

In response, Greg arranged for a neighbor to stay with his mother overnight. Having a sleep-in attendant boosted Greg's confidence, but not Carla's.

"Greg, the woman is even older than your mom. What if something happens to her? What if something happens to both of them? Have you thought about that?"

"No," Greg admitted. "I guess I haven't planned that far ahead."

Commuter Crises

Nobody plans to be a caregiver, much less a long-distance one. In the back of our minds is the vague idea that our parents will live forever in perfect health. Denial? Whatever the reason, caregiving takes most of us more or less by surprise. All of the sudden, we're saddled with a demanding responsibility we hadn't asked for and never wanted. The results can be stressful.

Stresses

Emily McLean's Aunt Julia was a childless widow who lived alone in one of the prettiest houses in town. It was stuffed with sixty years' worth of furniture, crystal, silver, clothing, jewelry—you name it. Despite her declining health, Aunt Julia saw no reason to leave her home. The fact that Emily had to fight crosstown traffic several times a week to hire helpers, pay bills, and keep the ancient furnace running did not bother Julia in the least. At ninety-five years of age, she did not realize that she was inconveniencing her niece. "I was responsible for two lives," says Emily, "hers and mine. And in the process, I was getting totally frazzled."

Emergencies

Ken Rogers took the phone call in his Wall Street office at 10:00 a.m. on a hectic Monday. "You'd better come right away," the caller said, a neighbor of his parents in Poughkeepsie, New York. "It looks like your mother's had a stroke. The emergency room people want to know what medications your mother takes and who her doctor is, but I don't know."

"Neither do I," Ken said, and then dashed for home.

Prospective caregivers—and caregivers themselves—are sometimes caught off guard by urgent medical situations. Suddenly, "routine" information is no longer routine.

Contingencies

It was 7:30 a.m. when the home health agency called Aubrey Porter at home. They had no one to send to her mother's house

51

that day because they were short handed. They thought Aubrey would like to know She lives in Cincinnati; her mother lives in Lexington, Kentucky, ninety miles away. She must have help to bathe, dress, walk, and prepare food. "I had no backup plan," Aubrey says lamely. "I had no idea what to do."

Financial Needs

"Family finances were never discussed within our hearing when we were growing up," says Joan Van Auken. "Now I have no idea what their financial resources are." Joan must arrange care for her aging parents, but has no idea what health insurance they have, whether they can afford a nursing home, or what financial assets they have. "They can't remember," she says, "and I have to try to find out. Can they afford a nursing home? Should I shop now for a nursing home that accepts Medicaid in case they run out of money?" Joan wishes she'd discussed these matters with her parents earlier, but they didn't think it was important and neither did she.

A Plan of Action

The Bible does not have a chapter titled "How to Care for Aged Parents." But it does have much to say about humility, love, and serving others. In discussing the obligation of Christians to tend to the weak and helpless among them, Peter cites an interesting reason for the purpose of serving: to be an example to others (1 Pet. 5:3). We are not being very good examples if we allow ourselves to be "frazzled" by the task, as Emily put it. But faced with a long-distance caregiving assignment, how can we avoid becoming overburdened?

Stress is to be expected. And so is the ageless comfort of the Lord. Throughout the Bible, we read of the Lord strengthening

His people. In each case, it was not their task that changed. Rather, God strengthened them in it.

"I did not ask for this job!" cries the caregiver.

"Be still, and know that I am God," answers our Lord (Ps. 46:10).

The "one who looked like a man" touched Daniel and said, "Do not be afraid. . . . Peace! Be strong now; be strong" (Dan. 10:18).

The prophet Zephaniah's words still ring true: "The Lord your God is with you, he is mighty to save. He will take great delight in you, he will quiet you with his love, he will rejoice over you with singing" (Zeph. 3:17).

Along with the Lord's strength, we can take some actions that remove some of the stress from caregiving. Before it gets to the critical stage when you have to drop everything and "do something," take some simple steps that will help to manage a caregiving crisis when it comes.

Gather Records

Allison Green flew home to Missoula, Montana, because of her father's critical illness. Allison lives in Baton Rouge, Louisiana. Her father called her to his bedside. "Everything you need is in my briefcase under my desk," he whispered. In the briefcase were copies of her parents' power of attorney, their wills and other legal documents, details of funeral arrangements, and the names and addresses of their doctor, banker, broker, pharmacist, accountant, and business associates. Allison describes it as "nothing short of a gift."

Whether your aging loved ones live far away or next door to you, one of the most helpful things you can do is to work with them to assemble pertinent information about their medical

53

and business affairs. Keep all of the papers together and readily available, perhaps in a folder attached inside a kitchen cabinet or in a conveniently located desk drawer. Keep copies of everything for yourself, and be sure that someone who lives close to your care receiver knows where to find this information. It will be invaluable in an emergency.

Assess the Care Receiver

Not all care receivers have the same level of need. Some need only a weekly visit to be sure that they appear to be well and are having no serious problems. For a fee, a professional case manager or nurse may be willing to visit with your care receiver periodically, assess his or her condition, and report to you. If the care receiver's need is greater, daily help may be required for cooking and housekeeping. Live-in help may be needed for some care receivers. Finding the right live-in person can be wonderful, but the situation can be disastrous if the live-in comes with personal baggage such as financial problems, emotional instability, or family problems.

Recruit a Local Helper

Long-distance caregivers cannot always be present with their care receivers and often have difficulty getting accurate information. Although it may be difficult, try to find a local person—such as a neighbor—to keep you informed.

Amy Young, a licensed clinical social worker who works daily with caregivers and their parents, warns that the most obvious choice, a family member, is sometimes the worst selection. Because of the close relationship, a family member may lack objectivity, creating tension among those concerned. "The most appropriate help is seldom the most available help," she cautions, and it may be expensive. "The biggest problem I run into is that people think that they can get suitable help for a 'small fee'" says Amy. That is seldom the case.

Finding someone to assist your caregiving efforts requires great caution. While a volunteer may help out in order to do a good deed, the quality of help may not be ideal. And some volunteers quit abruptly. Although their contributions may be valuable, be cautious about depending on volunteers entirely.

If your assistant is to be compensated, it is best to be as thorough in hiring them as you would for any job. Remember that "nice" people may not be what they seem; these same nice folk may walk off with the family silver. When hiring help, spell out the job description. Review the care receivers' homeowner's insurance policy to be certain paid workers in the home are covered. In any event, be sure that good liability coverage is in place in case a helper in the home, paid or volunteer, is injured. You may need workman's compensation insurance, depending upon how many workers you have and how many hours they work. Consult an insurance professional for answers.

A caregiver working in a private home should be bonded. Even when bonded caregivers are used, professionals advise removing portable items of value from the house, including such things as silverware, computers, small appliances, and handmade quilts. Before hiring, make a complete inventory of household items. The importance of working out an accountability agreement before hiring a live-in attendant—or even one who comes to the home regularly but does not spend the night—cannot be overemphasized.

All caregivers, paid or volunteer, will need local supervision. If you are not able to be on site regularly, you will need to find someone locally to keep tabs on the help, and finding such a supervisor may not be easy.

Sort Out Financial Issues

Financial issues are the bane of caregiving. Understanding them is critical for providing adequate care and averting a crisis. Medicare, the government health insurance program for the elderly, generally begins coverage at age sixty-five, so it is the primary insurer for most aging parents. But it's not a cure-all. Medicare pays for very little in-home support or nursing home care.

Many elderly people have secondary insurance that pays after Medicare. Some have long-term care insurance. If your care receiver has few resources, he or she may qualify for Medicaid, the government health insurance program for the poor.

It may be well worth what it costs to discuss your parents' finances with a lawyer who specializes in elder care. Buying an hour of a professional expert's time may save you and your parents money in the long run.

Look after Household Business

Day-to-day financial transactions need attention also. When balancing his parents' checkbook, Frank Perkins discovered his father, Harry, was writing a lot of checks to "cash." *Why does Dad need so much cash?* Frank wondered. A little sleuthing revealed that the man who cut the grass, realizing that Harry's memory was failing, was in the habit of collecting his pay two or three times a week. Harry never remembered that the man had already been paid.

Although many elderly persons are able to take financial responsibility, others cannot. One solution is to provide a box where care receivers can drop receipts, bills, bank statements, tax notices, and other important documents. The caregiver can collect the contents of the box on weekly or monthly visits and be sure that bills are paid. Some bills can be routed directly to the caregiver.

When balancing checkbooks, be aware that the care receiver may have an ATM card, and watch for transactions not recorded in the register. Also be on the lookout for forged checks or evidence that your care receiver has fallen victim to a scam. Fundraising appeals and magazine subscription sales are commonly targeted at elderly people. Be sure to review the care receiver's accumulated mail.

Obtain a Power of Attorney

Early in your caregiving experience, obtain a power of attorney from your care receiver, or be sure that one is assigned to a responsible person. The person holding the power of attorney will have broad powers to act for the care receiver if that person is unable to make his or her wishes known. These powers may or may not include the ability to make health care decisions, depending on the wording of the document. If this document is not in place, a government agency or court of law may become the decision maker. (See the Glossary of Caregiving Terms for more information.)

Preplan for Emergencies

As Greg Marler points out, strokes and other emergencies happen fast. A fall or heart attack can instantly change your care receiver's life—and yours. Independent people can become dependent in a moment's time.

Plan for emergencies before they happen. Try to determine your parents' preferences among hospitals, assisted living facilities, or nursing homes before they have need for them. And have a response plan in place. "If you are a long-distance care-giver," said Greg, "you need a reliable car and a cell phone." Greg also recommends preplanning arrangements for responsibilities that may have to be shifted on short notice, such as child care, job assignments, and tending to household details like mail delivery in case of an unplanned absence. "You may have to leave with little warning," he says, speaking from experience.

Formulate a Long-Term Plan

Most long-distance caregivers could have seen their situation taking shape but simply failed to notice. If you can do so, persuade your aging parents to move closer to you while they are still well and active enough to make new friends. Make it clear that you want to involve them in a new life, not simply uproot them from their old one. Be sure that your care receivers understand their options when considering a move. Check the descriptions of available services listed in the Glossary of Caregiving Terms, and make certain your parents know what each means. Let them know that it is their decision and that you will support them, whatever they choose. Remember that any move must be made for the care receiver's benefit, not solely for the caregiver's convenience.

Finding Him Faithful

After six years of commuting between Fort Collins and Pueblo, Greg Marler arranged to move both of his parents to the same nursing home in Fort Collins, only a mile and a half from Greg's home. His father, still paralyzed from the stroke, is almost completely blind and deaf. His mother needs constant nursing care. Greg and Carla are saddened by the changes in their parents' lives but relieved that they are being cared for. They realize that the change benefits the entire family.

Greg's daughter, Kelli, explains. "While this is painful in a lot of ways because it means moving my grandmother away from the family place, it will be such a blessing to have them close by, finally. My Dad has made *many* rushed trips in the middle of the night when the nursing home has called. It's better this way."

For his part, Greg has come to know firsthand the power of prayer. "I prayed a lot during those years," he says, "and God is faithful."

Indeed, our Lord does not leave His children hanging in thin air. He has a solution for every problem. In Greg and Carla's case, it took a while. But, as Peter reminds us, when you turn your anxiety over to the Lord, you are giving it to Someone who cares about you (1 Pet. 5:7).

Chapter Five

Polish Those Clubs Again, Dad
Identifying Creative Nursing Solutions

Distance Dilemma	Dealing with dementia.
Caregiver Connection	Daily time alone with God equips caregivers for their exhausting duties.

Pauline Reynolds was a twenty-year-old nursing student when her father had an accident that left him temporarily paralyzed from the waist down.

"I'll drop out of school and take care of you," Pauline offered.

"No," he father said flatly. "You finish your education."

"But it'll be too much for you and mom."

"We'll be fine," Les Reynolds insisted. "Someday we may need a nurse in the family."

Forty years later, events proved him right.

While a student at Northwestern University, Pauline met Josh Gibson, a pharmacy student. They married soon after graduation and found good jobs in Memphis, Tennessee, more than an eight-hour drive from Pauline's hometown of

Evanston, Illinois. After the birth of their third son, Pauline became a stay-at-home mom. The years ticked by, and the boys grew up and started careers of their own. Pauline revived her nursing skills, and she and Josh accepted a medical missions assignment at Tenwek hospital in the Bonet district of Kenya, Africa, about one hundred and forty miles west of Nairobi.

"It was difficult financially," Pauline recalls. "We had both a house payment and a car loan, and the mission society only had money to provide us with one-way tickets to Africa." But the Lord supplied their needs. Josh became the first pharmacist the hospital had ever had, and Pauline's nursing skills were put to good use. "The conditions were unlike anything I'd ever seen in the United States," she says. "We worked night and day."

After two terms of mission service, the Gibsons returned to Memphis, where eight hours of driving time still separated them from Pauline's aging parents. One day the phone rang; it was Pauline's mother, Peggy.

"Your Dad wandered away from the house today and got lost," she said, trying to sound as casual as possible. "One of the neighbors noticed him standing on the corner and brought him home."

Pauline hung up the telephone, her mind whirling. The last time she visited Evanston, she had noticed several little things about Dad that seemed unusual. "One evening he became so agitated that he wouldn't sit down," Pauline remembers. As a nurse, she had recognized the early signs of dementia, but as a daughter, she'd wanted to ignore them.

"Mom needs help," she worried aloud to Josh. "But they have no money to hire anyone." She knew her mother well enough to realize that she would want to keep Dad at home. Les Reynolds had long since recovered from the paralysis. Now his mobility was part of the problem.

"If he is going to be a wanderer, your mom will need help twenty-four hours a day," Josh observed.

"I know," said Pauline, thinking about the five hundred miles of highway between Memphis and Evanston. "What are we going to do?"

Dealing with Dementia

"At first the changes in personality were so slight we didn't spend a lot of time thinking about them," said Sally Rutherford. "When we visited in June, Dad did a few odd things, but we chalked them up to normal aging. By the time we came back for Christmas, it was obvious that something was wrong . . . he just wasn't my Daddy anymore."

That scenario is typical. Dementia is a condition that advances by degrees, slowly robbing its victim of abilities. Loved ones respond with denial, hoping that the symptoms are isolated or will remain mild. By the time it is taken seriously, dementia may have robbed its victim of memory, decision making ability, and personality, leaving a complete stranger in their place. When that happens, a cascade of emotions are released in friends and loved ones.

Fear

"I sent him to the grocery one day to get a head of lettuce," said Lucille, "and he came home with three heads of cabbage." Those cabbages were enough to break the back of denial in Lucille. "I knew then that we were dealing with Alzheimer's disease or something like it," she says. That realization led to a horrifying conclusion. "I panicked," Lucille now admits. *He's losing his mind!* I thought. *How will I ever take care of him?*

When it becomes obvious that a loved one is afflicted with dementia, the questions come fast and furious—

- Will he know me?
- How will I take care of her?
- What's next? Feeding? Diapers?

Fear and panic are typical responses to new and unsettling situations. When that situation involves the mind of a loved one, the emotions are even more intense.

Grief

Caregiving for dementia patients brings some of the frustrations of caring for a toddler. The care receiver lacks judgment, communicates poorly, and may even throw tantrums. Unlike caring for a healthy child, caregiving for a dementia patient lacks the reward of watching developmental milestones fly by and the satisfaction of seeing the child grow into productive adulthood. Instead, the caregiver witnesses a depressing, downhill slide toward utter disability and, finally, the release of death. For caregivers to experience depression under those circumstances is not unusual or abnormal. Caregivers for dementia patients often grieve long before the patient dies.

"When I had to put my mother in a nursing home, I cried for four days," said Gail. "When she died, I didn't shed a tear. Her death was an anticlimax. I had already grieved."

Danger

One night Marjorie walked into the kitchen of her suburban Pittsburgh home just as her husband, Martin, was about to drink a cup of coffee. Martin had never been violent toward his wife or anyone else; but with dementia gripping his mind, he lost control of his emotions, grabbed his wife by the collar and heaved her out the front door. He shut the door and locked it, then sat down to enjoy his coffee. When he'd finished, he unlocked the door and let her back in, remarking pleasantly that he had not wished to have an audience for his coffee break.

"After that bizarre incident," said Marjorie, "I began to carry my house key in my pocket most of the time."

Marjorie's experience reveals an unsettling but practical aspect of caring for adults with dementia—the need for physical precautions. Unlike an uncooperative toddler, the senile adult is too big to pick up and carry to his room. And unlike a child, a senile adult is capable of doing great harm by acting out in anger or frustration. Women taking care of bigger, stronger husbands are particularly at risk, even when the care receiver has no history of aggressive behavior.

Exhaustion

Caring for a dementia victim is draining physically because routine daily activities present major—and time-consuming—challenges. Michelle lives in San Diego. She starts her day at 6:15 a.m. by waking her mother, who lives with Michelle and her husband. She spends the next three hours helping her mother shower, dress, and eat breakfast. Michelle drives her mom to an adult day care center by 9:15 a.m. Then Michelle, who runs a business out of her home, begins her own workday.

Lucille (whose husband brought home the load of cabbages) found that as her husband's Alzheimer's disease progressed, he seemed to forget how to feed himself. "Did you ever try to feed a baby who wasn't very hungry?" she asks. "You can waste even more time trying to feed an adult who doesn't want to eat." She mentions another fact of life that dementia caregivers usually face: incontinence. "If you think it is a lot of work to keep a toddler in clean pants, try diapering a full-grown adult," Lucille says ruefully.

Even when the care receiver lives at a skilled nursing facility, the routine can be exhausting. Family caregivers often assist by feeding at some meals or doing laundry. Even if the family member merely visits to provide presence and "check on Mom," the added activity can become an exhausting addition to an already crowded daily or weekly schedule.

Through all the challenges of caring for a dementia patient—especially over distance—the person whose needs may go unmet is the caregiver him- or herself.

Recharging One Day at a Time

Where does continuing strength, both of body and spirit, come from for caregivers who face the never-ending demands of caring for a dementia patient?

Long ago, the people of ancient Israel discovered that their daily sustenance, the manna provided by God for food, came from heaven every morning and had to be gathered in family-sized lots each day (see Exod. 16:14–18). As day followed day, the manna appeared as regularly as the sunrise. That provision was intended as an object lesson for God's people. He can be trusted. What He promises, He will do.

Centuries later the prophet Jeremiah applied the manna principle spiritually when he wrote that God's love and compassion "are new every morning" and added, "Great is your faithfulness" (Lam. 3:23). "Give us today our daily bread," Jesus taught in His model prayer for believers (Matt. 6:11). As has been true for God's people over the centuries, long-distance caregivers find that God provides spiritual and emotional strength for His people one day at a time.

A little further into the same discourse in which Jesus teaches us to ask for bread daily, He adds, "Therefore do not worry about tomorrow, for tomorrow will worry about itself. Each day has enough trouble of its own" (Matt. 6:34). He might have had caregivers specifically in mind, for their days are as unpredictable as a teenager in a shoe store.

"Every caregiver has days that seem a week long," says Marjorie, whose husband locked her out of the house while he drank coffee. "Jesus' teaching about worrying about one day at a time is such a blessing to me. When I get into bed at night, I say to Him, 'That is the end of that, Lord. You and I can take it from the top in the morning.'" Caregivers must learn to close the door on each day, releasing its frustrations and failures to God's grace. His mercies really are new each morning.

So how do we appropriate that grace for ourselves? If God wants to supply our need of emotional and physical energy, how do we plug in to His supply of comfort, power, and ingenuity?

While God provided manna to the Israelites, they had to go out and gather it each morning. If they did not do so in a timely manner, it disappeared (Exod. 16:21). In the same way, we get our daily spiritual bread by shoehorning some time with God into our busy schedules. We must make time each day for Bible reading and prayer. This discipline is extremely important for caregivers, no matter how impossible the demands of their lives may seem. Without this daily time of refreshing, we quickly lose touch with the Lord. Just as straggling Israelites found that the day's supply of manna would disappear if not gathered, so we will find that God's blessings cannot be stored up for tomorrow; we must find them each day. If we do not make time for God's word each day, we risk going spiritually hungry that day, left on our own to face the emergencies that are bound to come.

Although the Bible does not limit prayer to any particular time or place, it gives ample indication that God's people have always prayed regularly. Just as we plug in our cell phones each night so they will be ready for use in the morning, so we must plug in to our power source each day.

Caregiving Solutions

The Bible speaks of giving thanks when you don't feel like it, offering to God what the New English Bible refers to as the "sacrifice of thanksgiving" (Ps. 50:14, 23; Ps. 107:22; Heb. 13:15). Sometimes the only solution for giving care to a dementia patient is to close the distance by making the difficult decision to offer the sacrifice of one's own or one's family's time.

Sacrifice

Living eight hours from Evanston and both working at demanding jobs, Pauline and Josh Gibson realized that there was no simple way to offer support as Pauline's father descended into dementia. Having no other family members who were willing to help and without adequate funds to hire nursing assistants, Pauline made a demanding and sacrificial choice. With Josh's support, she resigned her nursing position and moved back to her parents' home in Evanston. Josh was left alone in Memphis while she assisted with the care of her dad. During the eight months that Les Reynolds survived, Pauline returned to her home in Memphis for a total of eight days.

"Being certain of what you need to do is not the same thing as finding it easy," remarks Pauline. "There were countless times when Josh worked fourteen hours, then drove eight hours to Illinois in order to spend just one day with me. We would get a motel room and have twenty-four hours together. Even then, there were occasions when our brief time alone would be interrupted."

There are times when sacrifice is the only viable option.

"It strained us financially," Pauline continues, "because the trips were expensive, and we had to help my parents financially as well. Needless to say, when I stopped working it cut our income." Fortunately, Pauline's husband was committed to the sacrifice also. "It didn't upset our relationship," Pauline reports. "Josh loved my Dad and respected him as a Christian."

Josh and Pauline found that God's word is true. For each trial, He provides the grace to bear it. Those who are called to sacrifice in order to care for a loved one will find God's promise no less true.

Be Creative

Relaxing in her Memphis living room, Pauline laughs quietly. "Some of the times with Dad were sad; some were funny. Once to occupy Dad I put some balls of yarn in a container and got him interested in pulling the yarn out and winding it up into small balls a little at a time." When Josh arrived, he asked his father-in-law what he was doing. Les Reynolds replied that he had no idea, but he was enjoying it. "When I came back a few minutes later," Pauline laughs, "Dad had Josh sitting there winding yarn along with him."

In dealing with dementia patients, it helps to be creative. Caregivers benefit from redirecting their patients' attention, taking their minds off of things that are inappropriate or agitating and directing them toward something constructive. When Pauline's father wanted to play golf, she did not tell him that the sport was now beyond his ability. Instead she said, "What a great idea, Dad. I'll get out your clubs so you can clean them and be all ready to play." For days he joyfully cleaned the clubs, not realizing he often polished the same club again and again.

Simple chores like feeding and grooming can be difficult when dealing with a dementia patient. Giving medicine can be especially challenging. When Les Reynolds refused to take his medicine one day, Pauline hastily folded a nurse's cap from a sheet of paper and pinned it on her head. With as much dignity as she could muster while wearing sweat pants and a paper hat, she bustled back into the room, looked her father in the eye and said in her most professional voice, "Mr. Reynolds, I am Dr. Carter's nurse. Your doctor says it's time to take your medicine."

"Oh, sure," said Leslie, swallowing the pills immediately. Then he looked at her with rheumy eyes and said, "You know, my daughter is a nurse."

Pauline remembers escaping to the kitchen where she leaned against the refrigerator and sobbed. "It was partly because that confirmed my suspicion that he no longer knew me and partly because my dad was dying."

Did she feel guilty about deceiving her father? Not at all. "I was part nurse, part daughter," Pauline says, "And the roles were painfully tangled." But she realized that creativity and humor were her best allies in coping with the loss of her father's mind.

Pray

As Leslie's condition worsened, it was necessary to hire an outside caregiver, even though it strained Josh and Pauline to pay for it. "I prayed very explicitly," Pauline reports. "I said, *Lord, send me somebody strong enough to help Dad at night, and a*

Christian. Then I asked around." Within a short time, a capable young nursing assistant showed up on the Reynolds' doorstep. The lady was a single mother of five kids, active in her local church—and she was six feet tall, weighing two hundred pounds! She was able to pick up Pauline's emaciated father and carefully lay him in the middle of his big bed. Her presence was an answer to prayer.

"Ask and it will be given to you; seek and you will find; knock and the door will be opened to you," Jesus tells us (Luke 11:9). Doesn't our Father want to give good gifts to his children?

Be There

Occasionally Les Reynolds became so agitated that nothing but his wife's presence would calm him. Peggy would sit down on the sofa beside her husband, and the confusion would disappear for a few moments as he put his arm around his wife of sixty years and sat peacefully. "Besides quieting my father," Pauline reflects, "it was a beautiful demonstration of the love and trust that exist in a long, Christ-centered marriage."

Presence may be the only gift one can offer to a dementia victim. Jesus left his home in heaven to offer His presence to us for awhile. When nothing else is effective, the caregiver can at least be there.

Learning to Ride

Caregivers, at risk for spiritual and emotional exhaustion, need to hear not only that God's compassions never fail, arriving like manna every morning, but also that God's protection is real. Jeremiah reminds us also that "because of the Lord's great love we are not consumed" (Lam. 3:22). God's great lovingkindness (another possible translation) protects us from

71

the total physical and emotional collapse that often overtakes caregivers

As children, we discovered that the way to learn to ride a bicycle was to get on and ride. Sometimes we fell off and had to pick ourselves up and try again. In the end, we made it. Caregivers find that trusting God works in somewhat the same way. The way to prove Him faithful is to get on the bike and ride, committing each day to Him and then living victoriously, one day at a time.

That's what Pauline did. "It was a lot of work," she says candidly, "more than I'd imagined. It was much more time-consuming to take Dad for a short walk when he was agitated or to coax him to drink a little warm milk than it would have been to give him an anti-anxiety drug." Caring for her father took endless energy and ingenuity, but Pauline remained grounded in her source of strength. She prayed daily, meditated on God's Word, and looked to him every day for renewed strength and compassion.

"God is faithful," Pauline says peacefully. "He really is."

Chapter Six

Games People Play
Coping with Manipulative Family Members

Distance Dilemma	Arranging care when family members will not cooperate.
Caregiver Connection	Caregivers must set aside their differences to put care receivers first.

Charlotte and her husband, Tom, were living in Raleigh, North Carolina, three states and eight hours of driving time from Charlotte's parents, Charlie and Ella Ruth Hospers. The distance was nothing more than an obstacle to family reunions until Charlie Hospers was diagnosed with Alzheimer's disease. Even then, Ella Ruth was determined to care for him at home.

"That worked well," Charlotte says, "until Dad started wandering." Given the slightest opportunity, Charlie would wander out of the house, headed who knows where. Ella Ruth, experiencing age-related health problems herself, was unable to leave her husband alone for any length of time.

Charlie and Ella Mae lived for a lifetime in the same house in Circleville, Ohio. In fact, three generations of Hospers had lived in that town. Charlotte, the first from her family to attend college, was the only one who had settled in another place. For doing so, she was seen as something of a traitor to the family, especially by her brother and only sibling, "Little Charlie."

In spite of Little Charlie's proximity to his parents—he lived only ten minutes away—he seemed unwilling to help with his father's care. Charlotte prayerfully yet reluctantly decided to move her parents to Raleigh where she and Tom could look after them. Ella Ruth was sad to leave the house and friends of a lifetime, but she realized the necessity of living closer to her daughter, a registered nurse. "Tom and I thought it was the best thing," Charlotte recalls. "And we thought everyone agreed."

She was wrong.

Several weeks after the move, Charlotte called her brother. "I think we need to get Dad evaluated, and I'd like to have you involved in any decisions about long-term care. Can you come down to Raleigh next month?"

Little Charlie's response was as curt as it was unexpected. "No, Char. You took them down there, now you're going to have to deal with them."

Charlotte was baffled. "Charlie, I thought you agreed that we should make this move."

"Nope. I think they'd be better off up here. I'd have told you that if you had asked."

"But I did ask!" Charlotte's voice betrayed her annoyance with her brother.

"I didn't have time to answer," Charlie said. "You just snatched them up before Mom could change her mind, hauled them down there to live with strangers. Up here, Aunt Lula and Uncle Buster could help."

"What about you," Charlotte pressed. "Will you help?"

"Maybe."

"If I bring Mom and Dad back to Circleville, will you stay in the house with them at night? Mom can't do double duty. At least that way, she could get some sleep."

Little Charlie agreed to the arrangement, so Charlotte and Tom made the trip in reverse, moving Charlie and Ella Mae back to their home only a few weeks after they'd left. As promised, Little Charlie, who was actually six inches taller than his aged father, took up evening residence at the Hospers' home.

"It lasted about six weeks," Charlotte says, still exasperated with her younger brother. When Charlotte called the house late one evening, expecting to speak with Charlie, her mother answered the phone. When she discovered that her brother had abandoned their plan, Charlotte placed an irate call to his apartment.

"It's just not working," Little Charlie said, seeming annoyed that Charlotte would expect him to stick with the plan. "Besides," he added, "it was your idea. I never wanted to move back in with them. I've got a life, you know."

"I was livid," Charlotte recalls. "There I was, five hundred miles away and helpless while my good-for-nothing brother lived just down the road from my parents and wouldn't lift a finger to help."

Charlotte flicked off her cell phone and slammed it onto the table. "You're worthless, Charlie!" she said aloud. "Absolutely worthless!"

The Name of the Game

The vast majority of family members work together amiably for the good of their ill or disabled loved ones. Siblings sometimes find caring for aging parents becomes an opportunity for personal growth as they work together as adults, learning to know each other better and developing a deeper bond of love and trust than they had known as children.

But that is not always the case. Sometimes siblings or other family members resort to petty game playing as they dance around caregiving responsibilities. In identifying some of these, perhaps we are justified in remembering Jesus' instruction to His disciples when He first sent them out to preach, "Be as shrewd as snakes and as innocent as doves" (Matt. 10:16).

Denial

"It was the usual caregiving calamity," said Carol, who lives in Detroit, four hours from her parents in the northern Michigan community of Alpena. "Dad developed dementia after Mom had a stroke." Carol pitched into the dicey decisions and hard physical work necessary to move her parents into assisted living, but a younger brother who lived in Alpena never found it convenient to help.

"I was nearly frantic running back and forth from Detroit, and he couldn't see that there was anything to do," says Carol. "I heard him tell a relative, 'Mom's doing okay. Carol has everything under control.'"

Carol called her brother's game "sweet innocence." A professional counselor might call it denial. Many family members refuse to acknowledge—and, therefore, to take responsibility for—what's happening in their care receivers' lives.

Selfishness

Sometimes family members refuse to take part in giving care to an ailing loved one because they do not want to upset their own routine. Gina has been the primary caregiver for Buddy, a mentally handicapped brother, for years. But while her husband was recovering from a stroke, Gina herself became ill and was hospitalized, forcing two other siblings to take a role in caring for the handicapped brother. "Now they're acting like martyrs," says Gina, "because they had to care for Buddy for a few weeks." She adds sarcastically, "Families are so much fun!"

Resentment

Charlotte, whose brother Charlie will not help with the care of their parents, strongly suspects that the real reason for Little Charlie's behavior is his contempt for Charlotte and her achievements in life. Charlotte not only moved away from the small town where her brother still lives, but had a successful career, traveled to Europe, and worked overseas. "I think he resents my accomplishments," Charlotte says sadly. "He seems to think, *If she's so smart, let her figure it out.*"

Jealousy

Serena, who lives in Milwaukee, Wisconsin, felt torn between tending to her terminally ill mother and the demands of her marriage. When she began spending several days a week at her parents' home, a two-hour drive from her own, Serena's husband, Sam, became upset, demanding to know how long the arrangement would last.

"As long as she lives," had to be the answer. She continued making the trips, driving some nine thousand miles in seven weeks during an icy winter before her mother passed away. Serena's husband never did understand her devotion to her mother. "It was very hard on our marriage," Serena says forlornly. "I kept wanting to shout, 'She's my mother, and she's dying! Don't you understand that?'" Realizing that her husband's apparent jealousy was rooted in fear—"What if she has an accident driving all those miles on frozen roads?"—Serena kept silent.

Poor Communication

Serena realized, too, something fundamental about men and women: they process grief differently. "Men and women are very different by divine design," she observes, "and I don't question that. Still, it's hard when your best girlfriend understands you better than your husband does."

That knife cut both ways for Serena and Sam. In addition to picking up extra duties in caring for their children and managing a busy professional career, Sam was also grieving for his own mother, who had been diagnosed with cancer several years before. "He just held it all in," Serena now realizes. "Women cry and get it out, but he wouldn't share any of his burdens with me. I had no idea why he was responding the way he was."

Control

Kimberly, a social worker who specializes in health care issues, tells of a case where two family members spent nearly fifty thousand dollars on legal fees to determine who would be named guardian of their father. "It's not that they loved the man," Kimberly says sadly. "The name of their game was control—control of the money, the real estate, their father's affairs." In the end, the social worker was appointed guardian by the court. Family members will go to great lengths to control what they see as their own best interest. "Families that fight exhaust me," says Kimberly wearily.

Grab Bag

There are as many reasons offered for lack of cooperation when a family member needs care as there are people. Evelyn said she could not help care for her incapacitated mother because she, Evelyn, was too sensitive. It hurt her too much to see her mother suffer; others would have to tend to her mother's needs. Bob said that since his brother had more money than he did, it should be his responsibility to care for their parents. Tamera resented any time and money spent on her in-laws because they didn't deserve it. "They never like me anyway," Tamera claimed.

Nearly every family is likely to have some negative dynamics. How is it possible to gain cooperation or agreement from siblings or extended family members who quibble and quarrel?

In the Shadow of God's Wings

The psalmist David says he earnestly seeks God "in a dry and weary land" (Ps. 63:1). David finds God, too, and tells the Lord, "Because you are my help, I sing in the shadow of your wings" (Ps. 63: 7). Only from such a vantage point can we find the power to adopt Paul's attitude in facing uncooperative people while planning for the care of aging loved ones. "Be kind and compassionate to one another," Paul says, "forgiving each other, just as in Christ God forgave you" (Eph. 4:32).

Betrayal or manipulation by a relative is not new. Remember Jacob's problems with his father-in-law, Laban. He had promised Jacob the beautiful Rachel for a wife but gave him the unattractive Leah instead. Then the wily Laban had the gall to barter an extra seven years of work from Jacob (Gen. 29:15–30).

How is it possible to move beyond acts of betrayal or manipulation by a family member? Is it possible to forgive when the offending party is the one closest to you? What spiritual principles can we call on in such circumstances?

Gain Strength from God

First must surely be the admission that we cannot move past perceived injustice in our own strength. David clearly demonstrates that theme in Psalm 63:7, with his beautiful metaphor about singing in the shadow of God's wings. In verse 8, he says, "I stay close to you; your right hand upholds me." That is, he will stay close enough to the Lord so that he can keep his balance. "I don't have to lose my footing every time someone throws a punch of betrayal at me," David is saying. Relying on God's strength, he is able to move forward.

Trust God

Second, resolve to stay out of God's business. Gina, whose brothers felt imposed upon by having to care briefly for their handicapped sibling, learned the truth of Paul's words, "Do not take revenge, my friends, but leave room for God's wrath, for it is written: 'It is mine to avenge; I will repay,' says the Lord" (Rom. 12:19). "I didn't want to ruin our relationship over it," Gina says. "Besides, they will have to live with themselves after this is over." She knew that God takes stronger vengeance than we are capable of. When siblings shirk their duty or cause friction within a family, they answer to a much higher authority than a brother or sister. Let God deal with those who need discipline.

Letting go of a grudge or anger is not the same as saying, "It's all right; I don't mind." Rather, it is allowing God to deal with the matter of justice. It is a great relief to realize that God will take care of us—and others—in the way that He sees fit.

Realize That It Is Temporary

Third, remember that while caregiving is a temporary stage of life, relationships with siblings and other family members last for a lifetime. Few family quarrels are significant enough to risk losing the friendship and cooperation of a sibling. It is often best, from a purely practical point of view, to continue bearing more than your fair share of the burden than to gain greater cooperation at the expense of a relationship.

Tend to Your Own Needs

Sandy applies what she calls the Oxygen Mask Rule in dealing with her manipulative parents. She says, "Flight attendants always instruct passengers to put on their own oxygen masks first before assisting others. That's what I do with my parents: I make sure my own needs are met, and that makes me less vulnerable to bowing to their every whim."

Caregivers who are trapped in the exhausting cycle of meeting the needs of others but ignoring their own will have a hard time moving beyond blame and resentment. When you feel better about yourself, it is easier to be tolerant of others.

Exercise Your Will

Finally, exercise your will to move beyond what are essentially meaningless and distracting quarrels. And that's exactly what it takes to forgive—an act of the will. That is not possible unless God's healing hand is upon you. Ask Him for it. Find forgiveness from God, then offer that forgiveness to others. Never allow the person who misused you to win a double victory by ruining your life.

Moving On

After the bitter phone call with Charlie, Charlotte realized that she faced some hard decisions. Without assistance from her brother and without the resources to move her parents for a third time, Charlotte chose to resign from her nursing job and move back to Circleville to care for her aging parents, leaving her husband alone in Raleigh.

"Tom was so patient," Charlotte says. "I'm grateful for his unwavering support. But even at that, it was a very long year."

Sometime during that grueling twelve months, Charlotte realized that her anger was doing more harm to her than to her brother, who seemed blissfully undisturbed by the effect of his actions on his sister's life. "I still don't think he gets it," Charlotte says. "But the anger was really eating at me."

Charlotte realized she was carrying a burden too big to manage alone and took focused, resolute action. She scheduled a session with a professional counselor to resolve the matter. With help, she was able to move beyond what she perceived as her brother's betrayal of the family and continue to love him. Happily, she found that that one session was enough to uncover the source of her profound anger and take healing action. And the psalmist came to her aid. "My soul finds rest in God alone," he says (Ps. 62:1).

"I have learned to accept my brother," Charlotte says. "My anger was extremely deep," she says, "but I was able to let it go." It wasn't easy, she admits, but Charlotte herself states why it was so important to forgive the callous behavior of her only sibling.

"I lost my dad, and I won't have my mom much longer. I don't want to lose my brother too."

Chapter Seven

He Was My Father
Honoring Problem Parents

Distance Dilemma	Dealing with eccentric care receivers.
Caregiver Connection	Caregivers must define the boundary between service and manipulation.

"My father divorced my mother when he was eighty-two years old," said Alice Newman Stuart. "They had been married for sixty-two years. He left, would you believe, to take up with his old sweetheart, the girl he'd been engaged to before Mom. He got in touch with her in Jackson, Mississippi, and she told him to come down. They were together for three weeks before she threw him out."

That sad event marked the beginning of an odyssey of long-distance caregiving for Alice and her husband, Jim, one that would end only with her father's death. "I'm the only one of five brothers and sisters who kept in touch with Dad," she says. "My brother thought he was crazy. I think my sisters just gave up on him—but I couldn't walk away." For the next five years, Homer Newman put his daughter's loyalty to every conceivable test.

After his old sweetheart threw him out, Alice flew to Jackson from her home in Minneapolis to find her father living in a cheap hotel, with no money and fewer options. Who would hire an eighty-two-year-old person? She helped him get furniture and a place to live. "But Dad was a complainer," Alice says. "He hated the apartment and was desperate to get out." About six months later, Alice and Jim moved Homer to an apartment in Minneapolis.

"He seemed happy enough at first," Alice reports, "and it was so much easier to look after him. I was able to stop by and check on him nearly every day." But the aging lothario still had ties to Jackson. After about four months, Homer announced that he had found a woman to move in with and would leave for Mississippi at 1:30 the next morning.

"Why 1:30?"

"Why not?"

Sure enough, the eighty-two-year-old set out for Jackson by car in the middle of the night. "He didn't pack anything," Alice recalls. "He left his clothes, his furniture, everything." Alice and Jim had signed a one-year lease on the apartment, for which they were responsible. Alice never heard what happened with the new girlfriend, but when her father sent an address in Jackson, she shipped his furniture to him.

The next few years were a spiral of downward mobility. Homer tired of the Jackson apartment and moved into a low-income high-rise, leaving the furniture behind. The manager of that complex called Alice sometime later. "He said Dad was 'unstable' and asked me to come and look after him. Did he think I would move to Mississippi?" The housing manager was sympathetic to Alice's problem, but said that her father had wrecked his car, lost his wallet, and was behaving so strangely that he wondered if he'd had a stroke.

"My father's behavior kept me in multiple turmoil the whole five years he was alone," says Alice. "I bought him new furniture three times, paid the rent on I don't know how many apartments, and gave him an automobile." Besides the erratic moves, Alice had to contend with Homer's obsession with two things: cars and women. "I think that stemmed from being jilted by his old flame," Alice reckons. Sixty years ago, she'd broken off the engagement with Homer because he didn't own a car. "Now he would call me every once in awhile to say he was getting married."

Alice tried to keep up with her father's capricious moves, but it was becoming more and more difficult. The trips to Jackson were expensive, especially on short notice. As schoolteachers, Alice and Jim were not living in luxury to begin with. And the chaos was placing an increasing strain on Alice's life. "Once he called and said he was moving in with a drug addict he met on the street," says Alice. "I told him not to do anything until I could get there." Alice intended to hop on the first plane headed south, but she called her sister first to let her know what was happening. The response was not encouraging.

"Alice, Dad's gone crazy, and I wonder if you have too. You've got to quit letting him ruin your life."

But I can't do that, Alice thought. *I can't just turn my back on him . . . can I?*

The Face of Turmoil

"The hardest part was getting there," says Alice about the dilemma of caring for her peculiar father who lived over one thousand miles away. "So many of the trips had to be made with little or no warning," she says. "It tore up my life." Never an easy task, Alice's long-distance care became a Herculean one because of her father's unpredictable, even erratic, behavior. Many caregivers face a similar, if less severe, challenge. Aging parents may become eccentric or senile. Physical illnesses sometimes manifest themselves in psychological symptoms. Siblings or extended family members who are substance-addicted present a unique caregiving challenge. In each of these cases, the caregiver faces the usual problems of caregiving, but compounded by these factors.

Unknown Problems

Alice wonders what her father's problem really was. Could there have been a physical basis for his unpredictable conduct? Had he suffered a stroke? Was it a mental illness?

Alice remembers a pleasant childhood, in spite of some stresses. Yet about thirty years before he left his marriage, when Homer Newman was in his fifties, he became "different." "They did some tests," Alice remembers, "and I remember hearing that he had a loss of blood supply to the brain—but nobody ever followed up on it."

Was that the cause of his later abnormal behavior? Alice isn't sure. "He did not have a loss of memory, but his reasoning was way off," she says. "My brother thinks he was mentally ill, but I'm not sure. He always knew who people were and where he was. And he was able to drive from Minnesota to Mississippi, a trip of more than sixteen hours, all by himself—at age eighty-two!" Alice can only speculate as to the root of her father's problem, but believes it would have been easier to deal with him if she had had some idea what caused the odd behavior.

Many caregivers labor against undiagnosed or untreatable psychological problems. What in earlier life may have seemed like stubbornness, whimsy, or eccentricity may later produce irrationality, combativeness, or aggression—real problems for a caregiver.

Strong-Willed Care Receivers

Suzanne's father, Oscar, was a World War II veteran who became mentally unbalanced as a result of terrible battlefield experiences. For decades he lived on the streets of Davenport, Iowa, his hometown. Oscar was jovial and harmless, surviving by the kindness of a local rescue mission and some restaurant owners in his neighborhood who had known him before he became ill. Suzanne and her husband lived an hour away and made repeated attempts to get Oscar to live with them. He refused, preferring the "freedom" of the streets. Suzanne assessed her Dad's circumstances and made the difficult decision to let him roam the streets he preferred.

Caregivers, especially long-distance ones, face a tremendous challenge when the care receiver persists in self-destructive behavior. Making choices for mentally unstable relatives is more difficult than it seems.

Disconnected Relationships

Mark, who lives in Little Rock, Arkansas, wonders if he is obligated to respond as faithfully to his own father's needs as Alice did to hers. Mark's parents divorced when he was eight years old, but that was not the greatest trauma of his younger years.

Mark relates: "One weekend my baby brother and I were visiting our Dad in a rural county about sixty miles from Little Rock. Dad got drunk and passed out. The baby toddled into the creek that ran through Dad's yard. I screamed for help, and a neighbor came, but it was too late. My little brother had drowned."

A jury convicted Mark's father for his part in his son's death, and the man was sentenced to several years in prison. "He's out of jail now," says Mark, "but he still can't get his act together. Now that I'm grown up, do I have any responsibility for him?"

It's a question asked by many caregivers when the relationship with the care receiver has been strained or broken. Does the Bible require us to stay on the job when the job seems impossible? Can we honor our parents when their conduct is incorrigible? Can a caregiver ever quit?

A Family Affair

God gave us the Ten Commandments as rules to live by (see Exod. 20). The first four concern our duty to God. The last six concern our duty to ourselves and to each other. God honors relationships, and He created us to live within them. We humans are hardwired to be social creatures, living together in various relationships, notably the family.

Although God limited His commandments to just ten, two of them are devoted to family issues. The fifth commandment makes the single point that children are to honor their parents. The seventh says that husbands and wives are to be faithful to each other. If the Designer of the home used 20 percent of His precious commandments to order the family, that institution must be very important. In spite of various efforts to dismantle it, the family remains the cornerstone of a sound social structure. Cultures disintegrate when they cease to maintain the sanctity of the relationship between marriage partners or between parents and their children.

When the Lord gave Moses the fifth commandment, He did not offer a loophole to the effect that we must honor our parents only if they behave well, either during our childhood or in later years (Exod. 20:12, Deut. 5:16). Family relationships are so important that the Apostle Paul wrote about them several times, notably in his first letter to Timothy. In this letter, Paul assumes a multigenerational society containing younger and older men and women, widows, children, and grandchildren. Paul observes that the reason children and grandchildren are to care for their kinfolk is that such fidelity repays the parents and grandparents for their work in bringing up the kids. Paul adds that it pleases God as well (1 Tim. 5:4). Paul is hard on those who don't care for their families, saying, "If anyone does not provide for his relatives, and especially for his immediate family, he has denied the faith and is worse than an unbeliever" (1 Tim. 5:8).

It sounds as if the Bible means for us to take care of our parents.

To what extent was Alice, the woman whose parents divorced after sixty-two years of marriage, obligated to protect her father from his own folly. How should she have proceeded? What could she reasonably have done to care for her father without destroying her own life? Here are a few suggestions that might apply to Alice's case or to others in which care receivers do not seem to merit the sacrificial labor of their caregivers.

Protect Them Medically

Alice's father may well have suffered from some form of mental illness. If so, it went undiagnosed. Perhaps the cost of one plane ticket would have paid for a medical evaluation to determine whether Homer's behavior was based in a physical or psychological ailment that was treatable. In attempting to care for someone, especially at a distance, health issues must be addressed along with behavioral or lifestyle issues. Often, the two are related.

Take Appropriate Legal Action

It is possible that both Alice, whose father made a series of irrational moves, and Suzanne, whose father lived on the street, could have had their parents declared incompetent by a court of law and committed against their will to a mental institution. However, there is now a great emphasis placed by the courts on individual freedom. It is not as simple as it might seem to have a person whose behavior is questionable declared incompetent. Nor should it be easy; freedom is not a thing to be lightly taken away, as Suzanne herself concluded.

Yet for the cost of a round trip to Jackson, Alice might profitably have spent an hour with an attorney, exploring whether or not it would be appropriate to seek legal action in the care of her father. This issue should be approached cautiously and with the good of the care receiver in mind, not the convenience of the caregiver.

Clarify Roles

Codependent is a term coined to describe someone who shares responsibility for the bad choices of another by enabling him or her to continue making them. At first glance, it appears that that term might apply to Alice. She chose to continue bringing pain on herself by her interactions with her father. She saved him, repeatedly, from the consequences of his folly rather than letting him learn the hard way. Yet the problem with seeing Alice as codependent is that we do not fully understand her motivation, nor do we know if her father was mentally competent. Seldom, if ever, should one question the caregiving decisions of another.

Yet caregivers are well advised to beware of a codependent relationship or allowing care receivers to manipulate them into becoming enablers. It may be difficult to distinguish between callous disregard for a care receiver and loving firmness in enforcing the consequences of their decisions, but sometimes that "tough love" is just what's needed. Caregivers need to define that difference and stick with it—for the good of their care receivers.

Evaluate Motives

Alice gives only one reason for helping her father: "That verse in the Bible that says 'Honor your father and your mother' is what kept going through my head over and over. That's what got me through." Alice seems genuinely unaware of a second motive: she enjoyed her father's company, craziness and all. "Everybody said that of all five kids, I looked the most like my dad," Alice says with a smile. "We had some great times playing golf together. The last time was just two days before he died."

While no one would begrudge father and daughter a friendly game of golf, that does put Alice's numerous trips to Jackson in a different light. Her motives were mixed. Her father's freedom gave her some freedom as well.

Caregivers typically must sort through a collage of motivations for doing what that do. That may be especially true when the care receiver exhibits behavioral problems. Caregivers must sift through their anger, denial, grief, selfishness, or greed to arrive at pure motives, which place the needs of the care receiver first.

Set Boundaries

If the question is "Do I have to help care for my crazy old father?" the answer would appear to be yes, you do. But if the question is "Do I have to let him call all the shots?" the answer is no. Caregivers have a right to control their own circumstances.

Counselors and psychologists talk about constructing personal boundaries. Sometimes setting a boundary is as simple as developing a mental attitude that enables me to give of my own free will rather than in response to pressure from others. Caregivers must set boundaries in other areas as well.

Finances. It is important to decide early on how much financial help to offer a care receiver. As caregivers must also care for themselves and are often approaching retirement age, they must consider their own needs as well as those of the care receiver. Enigmatic care receivers require even greater discernment in this area because their poor decisions can have a financial impact on the caregiver.

Responsibility. Care receivers sometimes wish to make others responsible for every aspect of their lives. They refuse to be responsible for their own decisions or their own care. Caregivers must determine which responsibilities their care receivers can accept and then insist that they do so. For instance, Alice might have benefited from setting clearer boundaries for her father by refusing to accept financial responsibility for his broken lease agreements.

Manipulation. Genuine self-denial, as taught in the Bible, is never made out of shame or under pressure; it is freely given. Caregivers might well ask, "Am I doing this because my parents are shaming or manipulating me into it, or am I making this sacrifice because I have chosen to?" Caregivers must enforce the boundary against manipulation; care receivers often push against it.

Extremes. Alice and her siblings seemed to believe that only two responses to their father were possible: ignore him or indulge him. There may have been a middle road, one that would have met his needs without tolerating his erratic behavior.

Long-distance caregivers face a tremendous challenge. For those involved with problematic care receivers, the challenge is doubled. But God's Word is entirely clear on what our responsibilities are. We must honor our parents.

After the Sound and Fury

Five years after leaving his wife, Homer Newman suffered a massive stroke and died. Those five years were a whirlwind of broken relationships, wasted money, shiftless moves, and foolish choices. Of his five children, Alice was the only one to maintain a relationship with her father to the end.

With the benefit of hindsight, Alice is able to see that her father's care might have been managed differently. She was perhaps too permissive of his eccentric choices, too quick to rush to his aid, too willing to finance his recovery from disaster. Like a doting parent, the child would rather have spoiled her father than alienated him. She learned along the way, and those lessons were attained through trials.

"It was a nightmare," she says bluntly. "I did the best I could to survive it."

But would she do it again? "Yes," she says simply. "What else could I do? He was my father."

Chapter Eight

I Forgive You, Mother
Repairing Broken Relationships

Distance Dilemma	Forgiving family members who have wronged you.
Caregiver Connection	Forgiveness is an act of the will powered by the Lord.

It had been a typical, unpleasant visit with her mother. Now it was time to leave, and seven hours of hard driving lay between the Knoxville, Tennessee, nursing home and Jimmye's home in Richmond, Virginia. As Jimmye left, her mother's petulant voice followed her down the hall. "I can't believe a daughter could do this to her mother. And you call yourself a Christian. I'll sue you for what you've done to me!"

Alma Keller could muster a strong voice for a woman in her mid-eighties, a stroke victim with a spine filled with fractured vertebrae. That voice had haunted Jimmye as long as she could remember. "Many a night I went to bed hearing Mother and Dad arguing. When I woke in the morning, they were already up and at it again." Often, they argued about who was to blame for Jimmye's birth.

"I never wanted another baby," Alma would scream.

"Then you should have done something about it," her husband would retort.

"They didn't want me," Jimmye says, still hurt by the realization. "That's why they gave me a boy's name. They were hoping that, if they had to have another child, at least they might have a boy." The child drew the bedclothes over her ears to block out the angry voices, but she never quite succeeded. "I arrived at adulthood believing that I was totally worthless," says Jimmye. "My mother had convinced me that nobody wanted me."

Jimmye grew up in Knoxville, the youngest of five children, three girls and two boys. The Kellers' home life was chaotic, to say the least. Alma and Ed Keller were married and divorced from each other three times while Jimmye was growing up. She now realizes that her mother was spoiled, a controller who always demanded her own way. She accused her husband of infidelity, something Jimmye knew was not true, and tried to draw Jimmye into the dispute. Whenever Ed Keller took his daughter to town, Alma rudely questioned Jimmye when they returned home.

"Who did you talk to?"

"Nobody."

"You know that's a lie."

Somehow Jimmye managed to grow up, go to college, and find Steve, a patient, gentle Christian who became her husband. They had two children. Jimmye had heard the gospel from her brother as a child and made a profession of faith at age seven. However, by the time Jimmye was in her twenties, she said she "had powered down" spiritually. One afternoon, filled with dissatisfaction over her marriage, her children, and life in general, she sat down in her rocking chair.

"I prayed, *If there is more, Lord, then take my life. Forgive me for sinning. Amen.* That was my total prayer." The prayer may have been simple, but the Lord heard it. After about twenty minutes, Jimmye reports, "I knew a transaction had taken place. I fell to my knees, burst into tears, and thanked the Lord for saving my soul." Jimmye says that the next day, "The grass was greener, the sky bluer. Steve was so sweet, and the children were all of a sudden perfect."

But one thing remained the same: Jimmye's bitter feelings over her relationship with her mother.

By this time, Jimmye and Steve lived about an hour south of Knoxville in the small town of Athens, Tennessee. Ed Keller had passed away, and Alma's health was deteriorating. One of Jimmye's sisters lived nearby and served as their mother's primary caregiver. "I drove up there about once a week," Jimmye says, "to be my sister's cheerleader." Those visits occasioned more painful interactions with her mother, according to Jimmye. "I was cleaning her house one day, and it was terribly hot. I thought I would die of heat stroke, but she refused to let me turn on the air conditioning or even open a window–I think she enjoyed seeing me uncomfortable."

After several years, Steve's company transferred him to Richmond, and the family moved. Jimmye now lived seven hours away from her mother and made the trip home only every four to six weeks. The distance became a kind of insulation against the emotional pain of dealing with her mom. Jimmye began to wonder if she really needed to resolve the old hurts. Maybe the pain would just go away.

But time and distance were no help Jimmye's life was wracked by anger and bitterness. "I began to wonder why I couldn't get rid of the old hurt," she says. Remembering how freely Jesus had forgiven her, Jimmye wondered why she was unable to forgive her mother. *What's wrong with me?* she wondered. *Why can't I forgive?*

The Wounds

Jimmye's story, unfortunately, is not unique. Many caregivers are separated from their care receivers by more than miles. Old and deep wounds may mar the relationship between parent and child, brother and sister, or members of the extended family. Whether occasioned by rejection, abuse, neglect, or some other mistreatment, childhood wounds can remain fresh for years.

In some cases, the wound is caused by rejection. Even wounds caused by someone other than the care receiver may affect the caregiver's relationship with the care receiver. "My parents gave me away," Lorraine says bluntly. "They divorced when I was four years old, and neither of them wanted me." It's not as if Lorraine's mother had been an unmarried teenager who made the courageous decision to put her newborn up for adoption in order to offer her a better life. Instead, they were reasonably well off adults who simply did not want the encumbrance of a child. "I got thrown out with the junk from the attic," Lorraine says bitterly. Thankfully, she was adopted by fine people, but the wound inflicted by Lorraine's biological parents remains deep. "It still hurts, after all these years, to know that they thought so little of me that they would give me away."

Often, the wounds are compounded by denial by the offending party. After her conversion experience, Jimmye tried to share her new, deeper Christian faith with her mother. "Mom," she began, "Jesus has filled my heart with His love. I . . . I want you to know that I forgive you for the hurtful things you said to me when I was little."

Alma Keller looked up, surprised. "I never did anything to you that needs to be forgiven," she said indignantly.

On another occasion, Jimmye tried to clear the air by gently pointing out exactly what had hurt her. "When you and Dad used to bicker about not wanting me," she told her mother, "that really upset me. In fact, it still hurts. But I love you, and now that I've grown up, I hope you have come to love me too."

Alma laughed aloud. "In the first place, Jimmye, I never did anything to hurt you. Even if I had, I wouldn't blubber about it now."

Is it possible to forgive someone who will not repent? Can a relationship be repaired when only one party acknowledges the rift? Can wounds as deep as those inflicted by a loved one ever heal? What is forgiveness anyway?

The Forgiveness Process

C. S. Lewis remarks in *Mere Christianity*, "Everyone says forgiveness is a lovely idea, until they have something to forgive." Recollections like Jimmye's and Lorraine's cannot merely be dismissed. Yet Christ taught that we must forgive if we are to be forgiven (Mark 11:25; Luke 6:37). Forgiveness—both received from God and given to others—is at the heart of our faith. Jimmye puts her finger on the starting point for forgiveness, reflecting on her own situation. She says, "I wondered why the seven hours of distance between my mother and me didn't help me see her attitudes from another point of view. In time, I realized that I was looking for a quick fix, but I began to see that forgiveness is a process." Here are some first steps for beginning the process of forgiveness in relationships between caregiver and care receiver.

Recognize the Cost

Forgiveness is a costly thing; it cost Jesus His life. To face the cross in order to cleanse human beings of sin took Jesus thirty-three years of earthly preparation, and even then He would have avoided the sacrifice if that had been possible. He did not wish to die, but He did so in order to bring our forgiveness.

Forgiveness is costly in human relationships too. To forgive requires sacrificing one's pride, giving up a claim to revenge, and laying aside the emotional leverage that comes from being victimized. These things are never easy.

Exercise Your Will

To forgive someone who has wronged you requires a conscious act of the will. Jesus joined his will with the Father's, saying "Thy will be done." For us to forgive requires a similar decision. It involves making the choice to side with God. This does not bring a warm, fuzzy feeling. Forgiveness is not a feeling at all. Rather, it is exercising the difficult choice to see those who have wronged us as God sees them and to wish for their eternal good, not harm.

In doing so, we are exercising the same standard to which God held Himself in forgiving us. Speaking from the cross, Jesus made it clear that He forgave those who could not have cared less about Him and His message. While enduring the torture that accompanied submission to the Father's will, Jesus asked the Father to forgive His tormentors (Luke 23:34). Whether they accepted His forgiveness or not is another question. For his part, Jesus forgave.

Be Patient

Forgiveness is not only difficult but is often slow, being accomplished over a period of time. The passage of time can bring healing because it puts the hurt into perspective. Over time we gain maturity, breadth of intellect, and widened horizons; we are enabled to release our hurts to the Lord and let bygones be bygones.

Joseph was seventeen years old when his brothers sold him into Egyptian slavery. For thirteen long years he served Potiphar and even did jail time before, at age thirty, he entered Pharaoh's service (see Gen. 41:41–46). One wonders if the lapse of time was not intentional on God's part. Perhaps he allowed those thirteen years to crawl by so that Joseph could begin to think of something besides revenge. Even more time went by before his bearded brothers came to Egypt to buy food. It is no wonder that they did not recognize their brother; Joseph was close to forty years old by then. Clean shaven, wearing regal robes, and speaking to them through an interpreter, the high government official who met with the ragged sons of Israel bore no resemblance to the teenager they had stripped to his underwear and sold as a slave.

Joseph's perspective, as well as his visage, had changed. The wrong done so long ago was no longer a wound, but merely a scar, left as a reminder of how far God can bring a slave boy. The wrong Joseph had suffered did not seem as important as it had twenty-five years before. Joseph assured his brothers that they now had nothing to fear (Gen. 45:5; 50:19–21).

Time—or rather, the maturity, wisdom, and deepened faith that come with time—heals all wounds.

Rely on God's Power

June, whose mother had always made a point of telling her she was ugly and untalented, states a universal truth: "Unless forgiveness is of the Lord and is flowing through you, it is very difficult, almost impossible, to deal with the kind of situation I had. Forgiveness must come from the Lord."

In our own strength, we cannot forgive. We don't have enough humility, enough patience, enough love. God must pour those graces into our hearts. If you are dealing with a difficult loved one and a deep, ancient wound, realize that you cannot forgive on your own. You must seek God's power in order to forgive.

Choose Freedom

To forgive others does not mean that you become their doormat. Forgiving a mean-spirited mother does not require trying to be the perfect daughter. Forgiving an abusive husband does not require submitting to repeated abuse. Instead, forgiveness brings freedom for the one wronged. And that freedom brings power, the power to assert one's will and take control of one's life. The act of forgiveness itself is an act that asserts power over the past. To use a vernacular expression, true forgiveness robs the abuser of his or her ability to "yank my chain." When we truly forgive, the victimizer loses rather than gains control over our lives. He or she loses the position of emotional boss. This unshackling of our emotions leaves God free to do great things in our lives.

Be Realistic about Reconciliation

"I thought that now that I was on firm footing as a Christian, I'd just love him to the Lord," said Sharon about her abusive husband. "After being shouted at and beaten up one more time, I realized I needed to get out permanently before he killed me."

Forgiveness and reconciliation do not always coincide. Sometimes an abused woman, having forgiven the husband who tortured her, thinks it is her duty to go back into the marriage. That is not necessarily so. Often such a woman merely puts herself back in harm's way. Forgiveness is always possible. Mending relationships, sadly, is not.

Like the partner of an abusive spouse, caregivers for unloving care receivers must sometimes face the unhappy fact that a happy relationship between them is not possible. In such cases, the abuse may be emotional, as it was for Jimmye. People like Alma Keller, drowning in self-centeredness, have no idea what they want from others. No matter how much is given, it is never enough. Forgive unconditionally, but be realistic about pursuing reconciliation.

Practicing Forgiveness

As Jimmye drove the seven hours home from the nursing home in Knoxville, she began to wonder, *Why am I doing this? To be yelled at by that bitter old woman?* Sometime later, she discussed the matter with an evangelist who held a weekend crusade at her church. "Get counseling," he said.

The advice went against Jimmye's grain. Wasn't seeking human aid with a spiritual problem denying God's ability to help her? Finally, she decided that the visiting preacher was right and entered the care of Dr. Harrison, a Christian physician who was trained as a counselor. Although she dreaded reopening the wounds, for two years she consulted regularly with Dr. Harrison, who helped her recognize the source of her pain.

"I wanted my mother to love me," Jimmye says regretfully "But Dr. Harrison finally convinced me of the truth."

"Jimmye," he said, "you must accept the fact that you will never get what you want from your mother. She'll never give you the acceptance that you are looking for. You can be bitter over that, or you can choose to forgive her."

"I realized," Jimmye says sorrowfully, "that I was going to have to forgive my mother without any hope of having a true union of our spirits."

So Jimmye began the process of forgiveness, and she did so by making the decision to forgive. Each day, whether seven hours away or at her mother's side, she would say to herself, *I forgive you, Mother.*

Deliverance did not come instantly, but it did come. At the sound of her mother's voice, Jimmye's stomach still churned. But as she continued to make that daily conscious decision to forgive, this unwanted emotional response gradually disappeared.

Jimmye's mother died several years later without any real meeting of hearts between the two, just as Dr. Harrison had predicted. But Jimmye, at least, had found peace.

"It is not the ending I would have preferred," she says, "but no matter what my Mom did to me, it is I who must answer to the Lord for my actions, not her. I am responsible for me."

And she is looking toward the future. "I have to move on," she says. "It isn't easy to forget the past, but I have to do it. It's an act of my will, and God has given me the strength to do it."

Chapter Nine

As Christ Loved Us
Caring for an Uncooperative Patient

Distance Dilemma   Dealing with difficult care receivers.

Caregiver Connection   We can love others because Christ loved us first.

"**D**o you know what those stupid nurses you hired did?" Diane held the telephone away. Her mother's screeching hurt her ear.

"Now, Mom," she began.

"They cut the tips off the asparagus and served us the stalks. Don't I stumble over enough ignoramuses in the street every day without paying them to invade my home?"

"Mother, please—" Diane began again, but the shaft had hit its mark. The crack about the nurses "you hired" stung Diane's heart.

"I'm going to lock them out!" Bang, she hung up the phone.

Diane knew her mother would do it, too. She would lock out of her home the nurses so necessary to her husband's care. She'd done it before. Diane's father, Chet Bailey, suffered from emphysema. The disease was so severe he was confined to bed. Twice before Carrie Bailey had locked out the visiting nurses, but Diane had been able to reason with her over the phone and she'd finally opened the door. But not tonight, Diane knew. Her mother was beyond reason.

Sitting in her office in suburban Washington, D.C., one hundred miles distant from her parents' home in Dover, Delaware, Diane knew that she was nearly out of options. She recalled the night her parents' longsuffering neighbor had telephoned to say that he'd called 911 because Diane's mother couldn't get her father out of the chair and into bed. She drove to Delaware that night and used time she could not spare to arrange around-the-clock nursing for her father. Keeping the nurses on duty had required a tug-of-war with her mother ever since.

"I went into trauma mode every time I had to drive up there," Diane says. "Mom was totally uncooperative and verbally abusive. She refused to delegate authority and let the nurses do their job without interference; she harassed them. That made it next to impossible to keep nurses—I worried constantly about Dad's care."

One night Diane became so upset that she suggested the most drastic alternative she could think of. "Dad," she asked him quietly, "do you want me to look into divorce for you and Mom? You need help, and I can't work around her anymore."

Chet Bailey stared at his daughter a long moment. "Okay," he whispered.

"It never came to that," Diane continues, "but that's how desperate I was. I was almost beside myself trying to arrange for Dad's care, and Mom hindered me every step of the way."

Diane looked at her watch. It was 4:00 p.m. From her office, she could see the Beltway traffic, already at a standstill. There was no way she could reach Dover in time to let the night nurse in. Reluctantly, she picked up the phone and called the Baileys' faithful neighbor, who had a key to their home. "Bill, it's Diane. I hate to ask, but could you let the nurse in when she comes tonight and talk Mom into letting her stay? Mom says she's going to lock her out, and I'm just about desperate. Can you help—please?"

"Can't," said Bill flatly. "They just quit. The day nurse came by to tell me she was leaving, and the night nurse won't be coming. Your folks will be alone tonight." Bill paused, letting the words sink in. Then he said in a firm voice, but not unkindly, "Diane, you're going to have to get more involved here. The nurses are fed up with your Mom. And with your Dad in bed all the time, I'm afraid your folks are going to get in really bad shape. They need you."

"I know," Diane said, fighting back tears of frustration. "But I just don't know what to do."

Roots of the Problem

"At best, a caregiver's life may be pulled in so many directions that it fragments," Diane says. "Mine was blown to smithereens." Diane's life was complex to begin with. She was married, had children living at home, ran her own business, and was a community volunteer. The time spent managing her father's nursing care from a distance was robbed from an already full schedule. When her mother began erecting barriers to caring for her acutely ill husband, Diane became frantic.

A lack of cooperation or even active resistance to care is not uncommon among care receivers. When the caregiver's nerves are already stretched thin, the situation can become explosive. Here are some underlying causes of resistance by care receivers.

107

Strong Will

Because parents or other care receivers are old and physically weak does not mean that they have become toddlers. They are still adults accustomed to making their own decisions. It is not surprising, then, that care receivers sometimes become uncooperative, angry, or resentful when they perceive that other people—usually those closest to them—are forcing them into dependent positions. Soothing such feelings displayed by someone who lives close by is hard enough. Distance intensifies the problem. Attempting to keep the peace and gain cooperation by telephone or through occasional visits can be extremely difficult.

Frustration

"She wasn't crazy," Diane says of her mother. "She was enraged at having an outsider in her house." That loss of control drove Carrie Bailey to bizarre behavior. "One time, she put hat pins in the sofa cushions so the nurses couldn't sit down," Diane relates. "She was angry because she had lost control of her home. Yet she would not—could not—care for Dad herself."

That frustration existed on both sides of the caregiving equation, as it usually does. Facing impossible demands on her time and patience, Diane remembers, "Every time I drove to Dover, I had real, physical symptoms from the emotional turmoil. Tears would be streaming down my face."

No one, not the caregiver and not the care receiver, likes the experience of caregiving. Frustration mounts on both sides as illness or disability robs both parties of a normal life.

Unresolved Conflicts

A history of prickly interaction with parents may come back to scratch caregivers as their parents age. Alan, who lives in Dearborn, Michigan, says, "My parents never approved of anything I wanted to do. As they saw it, I was a bad son for not staying at home and taking over the family business. Then when I married someone they did not handpick for me, they wrote me off." The tension between Alan and his parents made it difficult for them to accept his direction as they grew older. The fact that he lived in another state and came to visit, as they saw it, only when there was a problem made matters even worse. "I resisted their advice thirty years ago," Alan observes soberly. "Now they're resisting mine."

The knife of unresolved conflict cuts both ways, as Andrea admits. "When I was a kid, everybody thought my mom was fun and wonderful. I knew better. I would have done anything to get away from her crushing words." Now Andrea is a long-distance caregiver, caught between meeting her parents' needs and haunting memories from the past. "I'm almost fifty years old," she says, "and I still can't stand to be around my mother."

Conflicting Priorities

"How do you make a choice between being a mother and being a daughter?" Marty asks. After several years of making long trips to tend to her father's needs, Marty's children began to fell the pinch—and notice the tension. "My children understood why I made all of those trips to Granddaddy's house, they also knew that their grandparents did not appreciate my efforts." Marty continued in her role as both at-home mom and long-distance caregiver in order to set an example of faithfulness for her children. But it wasn't easy. "Good example or not," she says, "driving all those miles only added to my sense of being torn between my parents and my children."

Financial Pressures

Almost any sort of household help is expensive; nursing care is even more so. Diane, attempting to provide adequate care for her bedridden father made the decision to hire nursing help—over her mother's objections. Before long, the cost became an added reason to worry. "I discovered that I had not analyzed my parents' financial position as thoroughly as I should have," she admits. "The cost of care was draining their resources rapidly." That financial pressure added irritation to an already tense relationship between mother and daughter.

Poor Coping Skills

Neither Diane nor her parents were believers at the time of her father's illness. As a result, she and her mother both had limited emotional and spiritual resources for coping with the fear and frustration occasioned by Chet Bailey's illness. Diane says, "I didn't have anyone to set an example, and the only plans I followed for coping with my problems were the ones I made up." Diane had never heard Paul's words to Timothy about putting "our hope in the living God, who is the Savior of all men" (1 Tim. 4:10). Neither had her mother. As a result, tensions that might have been eased by dependence upon God were allowed to escalate. Diane prayed by instinct without knowing that a personal relationship with God is possible through Christ.

Loving as Christ Loves

Is it possible to love those who are unlovely? Can we rise above our baser inclinations and treat others as we would like to be treated rather than as they deserve? The Apostle John thinks so. He states the general principle upon which all Christian love for others is based in 1 John 4:11: "Dear friends, since God so loved us, we also ought to love one another." In our own strength we cannot love those who are unlovable. Our hope for loving others lies in the love that Jesus showed to us. We love them because He first loved us.

John guides us to this conclusion through a series of teachings. John notes first that we prove our love for God by obeying His commandments (1 John 2:3–6). Next, he points out that Jesus' love for us was manifested in action, not just words. Our greatest need was deliverance from our sins. Christ demonstrated his love for us by doing what was necessary to achieve that—dying in our place (1 John 3:16). We cannot die for the sins of another, as Christ did for us, but we can imitate Christ's love by taking action to help others. That action might include giving gifts of money or material, serving others, or doing acts of compassion to those in need around us (1 John 3:17).

In 1 John 3:23, John says that the two great imperatives of our faith are to believe in Jesus Christ, God's Son, and to love one another. According to John, that is both as simple and as difficult as this: God loved us even when we were unlovable; therefore, we should love others in the same way. We are to look out at others through His eyes and love them with His strength, in spite of the challenges that they present to us.

Following John's thinking, then, we are to love our parents by caring for them even when they are angry with us. We are to treat our spouses with dignity, even if we suspect that they are falling out of love with us. We are to provide for our children, even when their dispositions are not congenial. We cannot confer a benefit upon God, for He needs nothing from us. But if we do love Him, we will repay His love for us by loving others.

Impossible? John didn't think so. That "Son of Thunder" became the Apostle of Love, and he urges that same love upon us. These practical steps will begin the journey toward loving the unlovely.

Dwell in Christ

If you are to love as Jesus loved, you must maintain a close connection with Him. John makes it clear that one motivation for loving others is that we are eager to obey God's commands (1 John 2:3–5). That implies that we have already come to God in repentance and received Christ into our lives as Lord and Savior. If we have not, then this is the point where we must start. It is impossible to show the love of Christ to others if Christ does not first dwell in your own heart. Have you come to know Jesus? Have your sins been forgiven and your life transformed by His power? If not, invite Him into your life today through prayer.

Accept Reality

Caregivers sometimes struggle in relationships with uncooperative care receivers—especially parents—because they retain a childhood desire to be loved, accepted, and affirmed. When the caregiver is an adult who was verbally or physically abused as a child, the desire for acceptance may be even more pronounced. Some find that the hoped-for acceptance never comes. Women seem to have a particularly hard time coming to terms with the reality that parental approval might not be given.

"This is where my relationship with Christ comes in," says Lillian, who has made the decision to care for her parents regardless of whether they appreciate her efforts or not. "I'd like to hear those words, 'Thank you, darling daughter. We're so glad for all you do,' but I don't expect to. As I drive to my parents' home, I ask God to make all bitterness and resentment go away so I can make good decisions for them."

Knowing that her worth and acceptance ultimately come from Christ, not her parents, Lillian is able to love them without the expectation of being loved in return. She has received that blessing from a heavenly Parent.

Focus on Action over Emotion

To love care receivers as Christ loves us, we must be willing to offer them love-based help regardless of how we feel about them. Remember that love is an attitude and an action as well as an emotion. Fix the right attitude in your heart and focus on right action. The reason we give to others is because Christ first gave to us. Our action has its basis in objective fact, not emotion, and it has nothing to do with whether the care receiver loves you in return. You don't have to feel warm and fuzzy in order to demonstrate the love of Christ to someone in need. Thankfully, Christ made this same decision, placing His will above His emotions in the Garden of Gethsemane, when he prayed to the Father, "Not as I will, but as you will" (Matt. 26:39).

Letting Go

Diane finally persuaded her mother to readmit the nurses to her home and was able to re-establish in-home care for her father, but Chet Bailey succumbed to his disease a short time later. That left Diane to ponder how she would cope with caregiving for her cantankerous mother if and when the time came.

About that same time, the Lord sent a woman named Marjorie across Diane's path. Marjorie was a mature believer who began leading Diane toward a relationship with God.

"Finally, in God's time, I confessed my sins, turned my problems over to the Lord and found Him as my Savior," Diane recounts. Her relationship with Christ gave Diane an entirely new outlook on life. She says, "The Lord filled my heart with a desire to win my mother for Him." That would not be easy because the relationship between them was all but severed. "Mom always hung up on me when I telephoned," Diane says matter-of-factly, "so I prayed that He would allow her to spend time in a hospital or a nursing home before she died so that she would have to speak to me again"

For seven years, Diane and her mother lived mostly separate lives. During that time Marjorie grounded Diane with sound Bible teaching, and she matured into a woman of strong faith. She would need that strength to withstand the most painful words she would ever hear.

On her mother's eighty-second birthday, the day after Mother's Day, Diane drove to her mother's home for a visit. Just before their parting, Carrie Bailey, still bitter over Diane's handling of her father's care and nursing a host of other perceived wrongs, said to her daughter, "I will hate you for the rest of my life, and I'm sorry you were ever born."

"I was crushed," says Diane. "But unlike the old days, I was now established in my relationship with Christ. I knew that I had worth, no matter what my mother thought."

Grounded in the love of Christ, Diane kept reaching out to her estranged parent. Not long after the birthday visit, Diane made the difficult decision to place her mother in a nursing home. Carrie Bailey was even more irate than usual. "I can still see her face as the attendants lifted her from the back of the ambulance when we arrived," Diane says. "She glared at me and said, 'I hate you.'"

But this time Diane was able to respond with kind words. "I still love you, Mother," she said, and really meant it. "I didn't say that in my own strength," she reports. "That was the Lord speaking through me. At last, I was able to see her through God's eyes."

Diane spent most of the next eight days with her ailing mother. It was a beautiful, God-given reunion. "I truly wanted Mom to find the Lord," Diane says. "I no longer held bitterness in my heart for her. God had taken it away."

Still, Diane was fearful when she risked opening her Bible to read to her mother. It seemed to her that God was directing her to the Twenty-third Psalm. Peacefulness came over her mother as Diane began to read, "The Lord is my shepherd, I shall not want." When she had finished, the elderly woman called out in a surprisingly strong voice, "More! More!"

"Do you want me to read Psalm 23 again?" Diane asked cautiously.

"Yes."

"I read it over and over," Diane says. "And she received it each time. And on the eighth sunrise, when she took her last breath, I was able to let go, and accept the Lord's peace."

Because of the love of Christ, Marjorie shared her faith with Diane. Because of the love of Christ, Diane found forgiveness. Because of the love of Christ, Diane was able to see her mother through different eyes. Because of the love of Christ, Carrie Bailey found peace before she died. "Because I had received love," Diane says, "I was able to give it."

And the cycle continues, because of the love of Christ.

Chapter Ten

Just One More Spin
Dealing with Unsafe Drivers

Distance Dilemma	Convincing care receivers that they can no longer drive.
Caregiver Connection	Caregivers mix compassion with firmness to protect unsafe drivers.

Judy Allison lives in San Jose, California, about five hours north of her hometown, Lancaster. A late-afternoon phone call from her brother, Dale, left Judy puzzled.

"You need to come down here," Dale pleaded. "Dad is driving again and I need your help."

"That's impossible," was Judy's first reaction. After her seventy-eight-year-old father, Clifton James, had totaled two cars in less than two weeks, his insurance company had cancelled his auto policy. Judy assumed that would be the end of his four-wheeled adventures. "Then I remembered the secret phone call," Judy says.

While visiting her father's house not long before, Judy had observed her dad locking himself in his bedroom to make a phone call. Judy, concerned about this unusual behavior, had listened on the extension and heard Clifton trying to arrange a car purchase.

"I blew up at him," Judy admits.

"You're never going to drive a car again," Judy had shouted at her father.

"The heck I'm not," was his reply.

For three years Judy had been a long-distance caregiver, alternating two-week stints with her husband in San Jose and her parents in Lancaster. Just one week before, Dale had gotten their mother into an assisted living facility, and they had arranged for daytime in-home care for their father. Judy had been thankful that her commuting days were over. Now Dale was pleading for her to make one more trip.

"He's gotten another car somewhere," Dale sighed, "and he's been driving around town."

"What could I do about it if I came?" Judy was so sick of the problem that she no longer cared if her father was driving around without insurance.

"You could help me get him admitted to a nursing home. Dad's gone crazy or got Alzheimer's—one or the other."

"Why? What happened?"

"He sideswiped a garbage truck," Dale said. "He gave the driver his business card, said to please call him at his office, then got back in the car and drove away." The car was barely drivable, badly smashed on the passenger side. "Now they've nailed him for leaving the scene of an accident."

Ron Judson, chief of police in Lancaster, had confronted Judy's father at his office and confiscated his driver's license. The visit from a high-ranking officer was not surprising because Clifton James was a well-known attorney in Lancaster, practicing law there for his entire career with distinction and complete integrity. Yet neither Dale nor Judy believed that the lack of a license would prevent their father from driving, any more than the lack of insurance had.

"All right, Dale," Judy sighed. "I'll be there tomorrow afternoon." She hung up the phone and wondered to herself, *Why does a great career have to end like this?*

Time to Shift Gears

Many care receivers, like Clifton James, have lost the ability to safely operate an automobile. Thankfully, some of them realize that fact. Chris Reynolds's mother announced on her seventy-fifth birthday that she was headed for the bureau of motor vehicles to renew her driver's license.

"I was petrified," Chris says. "Mom had been losing mental capacity for several months. I knew she shouldn't be driving."

So did Chris's mom. Upon returning home with a shiny new North Carolina operator's license, she voluntarily surrendered it to Chris. "I just wanted to prove I could still do it," she said. "But I'm not really comfortable driving. You can sell the car now."

Most caregivers aren't so lucky. The saga of the car keys is played out in many families as caregivers try to convince their aging parents that they are no longer able to drive safely. This issue can be one of the most delicate—and important—that a caregiver faces. Why all the fuss about the car? There are several reasons.

Emotional Attachments

Most automobiles contain a part not listed in any dealer's service manual: the emotional module. Americans have a longstanding love affair with their automobiles. To most teenagers, acquiring a driver's license is a rite of passage toward adulthood. Though many of us will not admit it out loud, we turn our cars into people, assigning personalities to them and sometimes even names. Cars can become coddled members of the family. The ability to drive means freedom and independence to an older person just as it does to a teenager.

Dependence upon Transportation

And we are dependent upon our cars. American lifestyle is based on personal transportation. The inability to drive creates a major problem, affecting the ability to work, tend to personal needs, and maintain social relationships. In a few of the largest cities it is not necessary to own an automobile, but most American families depend on each member having a motor vehicle available to him or her. Those who cannot drive quickly become isolated and dependent.

Denial

To be forced to quit driving when you have lived all of your life with the twin ideas that cars are indispensable and lovable is a stunning blow, especially if you believe you are still a good driver. Aging people seldom realize—or care to realize—that their abilities are deteriorating. Many see the suggestion that they are unable to drive as condescending and insulting. While a few voluntarily stop driving when they become uncomfortable with their ability to control an automobile, many others must be confronted with evidence of their declining skill. Most limit their driving or stop driving altogether.

Distance

Like every other aspect of caregiving, this issue is complicated by distance. Caregivers who do not see their care receivers every day or even every week have a difficult time assessing their abilities. "I'd been going up to Mom's maybe once a month," says Bruce. "But her poor driving never came to my attention because I always did the driving when I was there. When she got into an accident, it really caught me off guard." Caregivers have a vested interest in maintaining the independence of their care receivers. As long as Bruce's mother was able to drive, the demands on his time were fewer.

Inevitably, however, the time comes when a caregiver must take action to protect the care receiver and others. Unsafe drivers simply must be prevented from driving. But how?

Steep Grade—Maintain Humility

One of the points Peter makes in his first New Testament letter is that we should approach others in a spirit of humility, "Not bossily telling others what to do, but tenderly showing them the way" (1 Pet. 5:3 The Message). "Clothe yourselves with humility toward one another," he says (1 Pet. 5:5). As commentator Charles Erdman says, "Humility is always an essential equipment for wide helpfulness." If you are faced with the challenge of confronting a driver who has become a highway danger, Peter offers solace later in this same letter: "Cast all your anxiety on him [God] because he cares for you," (1 Pet. 5:7).

All of the various English translations of that verse convey the idea that God's care is incredibly personal. "Unload all your worries on to him," says the Jerusalem Bible, "since he is looking after you." "You can throw the whole weight of your anxieties upon him, for you are his personal concern," reads the Phillips Modern English. "For you are his charge," adds the New English Bible.

Peter was not expressing a new idea. He was, in fact, quoting Psalm 55:22, written about one thousand years before Peter lived. The Amplified Bible translates that verse this way: "Cast your burden on the Lord [releasing the weight of it] and He will sustain you; He will never allow the [consistently] righteous to be moved—made to slip, fall or fail."

You matter to God. You really do. The feelings of your struggling care receiver matter also. We are brought back, as we are so often as caregivers, to Paul's admonition to the Ephesian church, "Be kind and compassionate to one another" (Eph. 4:32).

How do those principles apply when someone must be forcibly halted from driving? Here are some suggestions.

Make Use of Authority Figures

Sometimes a person with some authority can speak more convincingly to a care receiver than can the caregiver. That is especially true when the care receiver is the parent of the caregiver. If a family doctor, lawyer, or trusted friend expresses the opinion that the parent should not continue driving, the suggestion may be taken more seriously than if it comes from the child alone—never mind that the child himself may be a lawyer or physician! The service of an outside person also removes the blame from family members for taking the car keys away.

Consider Removing the Keys but Not the Car

Some care receivers are willing to quit driving if they can find someone to drive for them. In those cases, it may be helpful to allow the care receiver to keep the car and assist in finding a part-time chauffeur. Teenagers with valid driver's licenses have been known to take sudden leaps toward maturity if entrusted with and paid for the task of driving an older person on errands.

It may also be wise to leave the car in place even though nobody drives it. Having the car but not the keys may make the transition to nondriving smoother for the care receiver. When the time came for Donna's mother to stop driving, Donna hid the car keys but left her mom's car parked in the carport. From time to time her mother and her housekeeper, who did not know how to drive, would simply sit in the car together, sometimes for hours, without going anywhere. Odd behavior? So what? Somehow it helped the woman cope with her loss of ability.

Be Honest

"We made a mistake," Elizabeth admits. "We just took Dad's car one day."

Raymond Warden's first job had been as a chauffeur, and he insisted on driving whenever he was in the car. "A longstanding family joke was that Dad would drive the hearse to his own funeral," Elizabeth recalls. So it's not surprising that when Raymond's driving abilities deteriorated, he was unwilling to admit it. Raymond never lost his ability to drive, but the onset of dementia robbed him of the ability to find his way or follow directions. He could no longer navigate safely, but he insisted on keeping the car.

"We had talked about what to do with the car," Elizabeth says. "Dad agreed that my nephew Paul could have the car when he was finished with it. Of course, to Dad, that meant the day he died."

But Elizabeth's sister was determined to both prevent her father from driving unsafely and acquire an inexpensive used car for her son. She sent Paul to the house one day with instructions to bring the car back. Somehow, he got the keys from his grandfather and did just that.

"When Dad realized what had happened, he was crushed," Elizabeth said. "Day after day Dad would go to the garage door and stand there looking for the car. There must have been a more humane way to end his driving career."

Caregivers may become anxious about protecting their care receivers from themselves, but should resist the temptation to be high-handed.

Be Firm

"We tried to reason with Mother first," said Bruce, whose mother had become an unsafe driver. "Her doctor called me and said she absolutely had to quit driving. We sat down with her and tried to make her understand, but she wouldn't accept it."

Bruce and his brother, Jonathan, made a careful plan, involving help from a used car dealer whom they knew. They sold the car, legally, to the dealer and arranged for him to pick it up late in the evening, after their mother had gone to bed. The results were predictable. "She was really mad when the car was missing," Bruce says. "We were all three crying. It was awful." But the painful scene did not alter their resolve. "Mom simply had to quit driving," Bruce insists. "We did the best we could to help her admit that, but when she couldn't, we had to do something."

Finishing the Course

Caregivers must sometimes make difficult choices, and few are more difficult than the decision to prevent a loved one from driving. Compassion and firmness are called for, and humility above all. If someone must be stopped forcibly from driving, prepare for a hurt, angry reaction, but work hard, as Bruce and Jon did, to formulate a compassionate plan of action.

In this case, as in many other caregiving situations, a caregiver might well look into the mirror and ask, "Why am I doing this?" The care receiver's safety—not the caregiver's peace of mind—should be the motivation. Even in cases when receivers seldom drive, their car keys remain a symbol of adulthood and independence. Without them, they face a different way of life. Caregivers should be certain that safety is truly at issue before forcibly halting their care receivers from driving.

Judy Allison and her brother Dale worked together to prevent their father from continuing to drive. After his third car accident, Clifton James's dementia was so apparent that they were able to get him admitted to a nursing home where, they hoped, he would have no access to a car. Clifton took the move remarkably well, but stated that he had one goal remaining in life. His ambition? To get his driver's license back.

Some old motorists never die; they just drive away.

Chapter Eleven

It's My House Now
Facing Legal Realities

Distance Dilemma	Helping loved ones plan for the future.
Caregiver Connection	Careful estate planning eliminates many heartaches.

Professor J. Wilbur Vincent looked exactly like you might think a professor of ancient languages would look: tall, thin, and angular, with a kind face that never changed its expression. He and his wife, Clara, had lived in Xenia, Ohio, ever since the professor finished his graduate work. They had left their native home of Lawrence, Kansas, fifty years before.

The Vincents had one child, a daughter named Mary, who was especially cherished because she was born after they had given up on having children. Mary grew up, went to college, and married a fine young man named Douglas, who graduated from the theological seminary where Prof. Vincent had taught Hebrew and Greek for many years. Mary and Douglas moved to the far away city of Birmingham, Alabama, where Douglas became the pastor of a fast-growing church. They had two children.

Years went by, and Clara passed away, leaving Prof. Vincent alone in their little house on a quiet street behind the campus. Prof. Vincent found it hard to live by himself, but he did the best he could. Mary and Douglas came to visit now and then, but as the children grew, it became difficult for them make the seven-hour drive from Birmingham to Xenia. Douglas's career in the ministry was prospering. There were lots of demands on the family's time, and all of them were important. Visits to Prof. Vincent became infrequent.

Although Prof. Vincent had retired from teaching, he kept busy. It was his joy to research, write, and publish articles in the scholarly journals that made known new information about ancient languages. He enjoyed the work, but it took energy. Even though he was "pretty well," as he put it, he knew that his physical powers were gradually failing. In addition, he had never been a handyman, and lots of things around his snug little house needed to be fixed. Clara had always tended to that, but now she was gone. Prof. Vincent wondered what to do.

Seeking advice, the professor went to Geneva Engelhardt, a pillar of the church they both attended. Geneva, who had Prof. Vincent's best interests at heart, listened to his concerns and then said, "Why don't you deed the house to Mary? Then you can live in it for your lifetime, and Mary will have the responsibility of taking care of things. When you die, the house will be hers, and it won't have to be tied up in probate." Geneva had no idea what probate was, but she had heard somewhere that it took a long time.

The advice sounded good, so Prof. Vincent deeded his house to Mary.

Mary was delighted. "Look," she told Douglas, "now we can afford to put our children through college!"

On the phone with her father, Mary did little to hide her enthusiasm. "You're getting old, Dad, and that house needs more care than either of us can give it. I'm selling the house. You'll have to move."

"But that's not what I want," said Prof. Vincent. "I'm just deeding you the house, not moving."

"Sorry, Dad," replied Mary. "I can't trail back and forth between there and Birmingham every time a faucet drips."

"But this is my home," Prof. Vincent protested.

"Not anymore," said Mary. "You gave it to me."

What He Didn't Know

We can commend Prof. Vincent for realizing that he needed an end-of-life plan. Unlike many persons, he squarely faced the fact that he was increasingly incapable of caring for himself. Most people don't like to think about the end of their lives, so they don't. They wind up with no plan at all. But Prof. Vincent, with a terribly flawed plan, was perhaps in even worse shape. His plan was a poor one mainly because of ignorance. Let's take a look at the mistakes Prof. Vincent made.

He Got Poor Advice

The aging professor did not realize that a friend who is a dear, honest, and earnest Christian is not necessarily the best advisor on estate planning. Faced with a variety of complex legal and financial issues, he sought the comfort of a friend, not the advice of an expert. When making an estate plan, it is essential to get competent legal and financial counsel. That will come only at a fee, but a reasonable fee will be well worth it. Unfortunately, aging care receivers are often unwilling to confront end-of-life issues and are often unsure whom to trust for advice.

He Underestimated the Problem of Distance

Some things simply cannot be done from a distance, and maintenance of real estate is one of them. Geneva Engelhardt and Prof. Vincent both failed to comprehend that Mary would incur certain obligations by owning the house as well as some privileges. Mary, whatever else she may have done wrong, at least realized that she could not tend to her father's affairs in Ohio while living in Alabama. Care receivers are often naive about the problems associated with long-distance caregiving.

He Didn't Have an Estate Plan

If Prof. Vincent had been asked if he had a will or if he had given someone his power of attorney, he probably would have replied that he did not need to do extensive planning because he had very little money. Arguably, the opposite is true. The fewer assets one has, the more carefully he or she should plan to husband those resources for use in old age. Estate planning is nothing more than planning the effective use of personal assets, whether they are great or small. Having a proper plan will make your money and property available to you when you need them and permit you to dispose of them at death for the benefit of others. A plan should be tailor-made to fit individual situations.

He Mistook the Character of Others

Prof. Vincent misjudged Mary. He might have known his daughter well enough to realize that she would look to her own interests first. He asked no questions and made the unwarranted assumption that he would continue to live in his old home. The idea that Mary might prefer to dispose of the asset did not occur to Prof. Vincent. If Mary had been more sympathetic in her approach, she could have suggested other solutions to her father. But that would have taken time out of her busy life. Not only did she want to avoid inconvenience, but she also wanted the money. It is not uncommon for care receivers to rely too heavily on the goodwill of those around them.

He Waited Too Long

Prof. Vincent's dilemma was building for a long time before he acknowledged it. Years earlier, when he was still more vigorous, the professor might have been able to manage the sale of his home and make a transition to a condominium or independent living community. By the time he was willing to face his problem, he had very few options. "People who do not plan," says Elsie Pendleton, the trust officer of a bank, "leave a mess behind." Sometimes, as in Prof. Vincent's case, they create a mess for themselves as well.

He Gave Up Control

Prof. Vincent divested himself of his chief asset, his house, in a manner that did not serve his purposes. By doing so, he gave up control of his circumstances. He had every right to control the house and financial power it represented; after all, his own money had paid for it. He needed to keep his home—or the revenue from it—in order to remain independent. The house should have been the cornerstone of his retirement plan. Instead, it became a building block in his daughter's financial scheme.

A More Excellent Way

For all of his mistakes, Prof. Vincent did a few things right. Paul told the Thessalonians, "If a man will not work, he shall not eat" (2 Thess. 3:10). The elderly teacher had been a diligent worker and had hundreds of well-trained students to his credit. Twice the writer of Proverbs points to the example of the ant as a hard worker who stores up his provisions and gathers food at harvest (Prov. 6:6–11; 30:25). Here again, Prof. Vincent had done well, for he had taken care of what he had earned.

What Prof. Vincent might have done better was to follow James's biblical advice on applying "the wisdom that comes from heaven." One quality of that wisdom, says James, is to be considerate (James 3:17), or, as it is sometimes translated, gentle. It seems that God wants us to make things as easy for one another as possible, while still observing His standards of ethics. One way of doing that is to create an estate plan, putting our affairs in order and providing adequately for ourselves, to relieve the burden on others as we become less able to care for ourselves.

Plan Legal Matters

Hazel, one of five children, reports that when her father was dying, he reminded the family of "the papers" that were in his desk drawer. He meant a packet containing his will, his power of attorney, his health care power of attorney, and other items that would be needed in settling his estate. Hazel said, "It was the most loving thing he could have done. We knew what he wanted done and the assets we had to work with." Estate planning benefits not only the care receiver but also his or her loved ones. If your care receivers have not made an estate plan, urge them to create one.

Plan Living Arrangements

Eric and Pamela had lived their entire lives in Erie, Pennsylvania. Their only child, Janet, had married and settled herself in Charlotte, North Carolina. Eric and Pamela were in good health, active in their church, and had a wide circle of friends. In spite of their hesitation to leave friends behind, they moved to an apartment in Charlotte several miles from where their daughter lived. "If something happens," they said, "at least Janet will be nearby." Their decision benefited Janet as much as it did them.

After half a dozen years in the apartment, during which they investigated local retirement communities, Eric and Pamela put their names on the waiting list for the one they had thought best. In about a year, a suitable opening came, and they moved. More new friends entered their lives, and they took part in some of the numerous activities the community offered residents. After six more years, Eric's health began to fail and their choices were vindicated. Janet and her husband were close by to help. By this time, their new friends had become old friends, a marvelous support group during Eric's illness and, for Pam, after his death. To Janet's vast relief, her mother, now alone, was settled in a sheltered place with emergency help available.

By planning for their future, Eric and Pamela both maintained control of their circumstances and kept themselves in proximity to their daughter.

Explore Options

Eric and Pamela carefully investigated each choice they made. When it became clear that they should leave their home, they visited retirement communities both in Erie and in

133

Charlotte. Well before they needed assisted living, they visited several Charlotte-area facilities. When they made choices, they were armed with information.

Prof. Vincent did none of that. He made the choice to deed his home to Mary without ever considering when or where he might move. He had no idea what options were available to him. Could he live with Mary? Could he find an apartment? Would he be happier living in Birmingham? Would friends in Xenia help him maintain his home? To his regret, Prof. Vincent never asked those questions.

Get Expert Advice

Prof. Vincent needed to see a lawyer, preferably one who specialized in estate planning, to help him devise a plan for a comfortable retirement. Geneva Engelhardt, no matter how well intentioned she may have been, gave him bad advice. He needed a prayer partner, perhaps, but he also needed professional expertise in matters of law, business, and real estate. A financial planner could have guided Prof. Vincent into a plan for maximizing his financial assets and minimizing tax liability. A social worker might have explored options for living arrangements with Prof. Vincent, helping him find a sensible plan either for moving out of his house or staying in it. A lawyer could have helped Prof. Vincent create a will and understand legal issues surrounding the disposal of his property. The lawyer might have helped Prof. Vincent establish a trust that would provide an income for him during his lifetime and then for his daughter after his death.

There is no one-size-fits-all estate plan. It is essential to get competent advice when creating a retirement plan.

Estate planning pays off. Christian families are not immune to power struggles, and in the absence of a plan, disagreements are bound to arise. If parents are considerate of their children by planning ahead, there is a benefit to both sides. The parents' wishes are known and followed, so there is less incentive for children to become angry with each other. As James says, "The wisdom that comes from heaven is first of all pure; then peace loving, considerate, submissive, full of mercy and good fruit, impartial and sincere" (James 3:17).

The Bitter End

It would be nice to report a happy ending to Prof. Vincent's story, but there isn't one. When the professor complained to his daughter that he had no place to live, Mary replied evenly, "Aunt Eliza lives in Lawrence. You could move back there and live in a nursing home."

"But I don't know anybody there anymore," said Prof. Vincent. "Besides, I'm not ready for a nursing home, and Eliza and I have nothing in common anymore."

"Whatever," said Mary. "But you can't maintain the house, and neither can I. Besides, Douglas and I need the money from the house to put the kids through college."

So it was back to Lawrence for Prof. Vincent. Geneva Engelhardt was appalled at the turn her well-intentioned advice had taken. Prof. Vincent's friends were equally disappointed by Mary's action. One of them was bold enough to call Mary on the telephone. "I never thought you would sell the poor man's house out from under him."

"It's not his house," Mary rejoined. And she was right.

Prof. Vincent wrote to friends from his new place in Lawrence, where he had been assigned a room with several other men. He had no privacy for his daily time of Bible reading and prayer, no place for his books, and nobody to talk with since his roommates suffered from varying degrees of dementia and the nurses were not interested in theology. After three miserable years, he died.

It is a shame that this long, happy, productive life ended in sadness and boredom. That might have been prevented if Prof. Vincent had faced his situation sooner, informed himself about his options, and hired professional help to form an estate plan. Instead, he painted himself into a corner with his ignorance, mistaken judgment, and unwise actions. A good life came to a forlorn end.

All of us hope our lives end like autumn leaves, dying with a beauty that brings admiration from others and glorifies God. It would seem that a part of that end should include the careful planning that keeps us in control of our lives for as long as possible and makes our wishes known to those who can best meet them.

Isn't that something we can all do?

Chapter Twelve

Do You Think Mom's All Right?

Selecting a Nursing Home

Distance Dilemma   Placing a care receiver into a nursing home.

Caregiver Connection   Careful research and ongoing involvement give caregivers confidence in a skilled nursing facility.

Amanda Parker and her husband, John, were living in St. Louis, Missouri, when John's father died. They invited John's mother, Louise, to move closer to them from her home in Wichita, Kansas. Because she was well and mentally alert, Louise decided to stay in Wichita, close to her friends and church family. "We respected her decision," Amanda says, "but we did wonder what would happen in an emergency—we were almost seven hours away."

Amanda and John helped Louise sell her suburban home and move into a church-owned retirement community in Wichita. The facility offered the usual three levels of care, independent living, assisted living, and fully skilled nursing home care.

Louise moved into one of the independent living apartments, but Amanda and John were assured that someone would check on her every day.

In spite of the facility's claim that Louise would be observed daily, Amanda and John discovered that Louise had fallen and had lain on the floor in her apartment for three days before anyone missed her. The managers of the retirement community moved her to assisted living and promised an increased level of care. The Parkers visited every two or three months, and Jeff, one of Louise's grandsons, drove over from Great Bend, Kansas, about once a month.

"Louise had a telephone in her room," Amanda explains, "and we called frequently. I always asked lots of questions. 'Mom,' I would say, 'are they treating you well?'"

Louise seemed to hesitate just a bit before enthusiastically answering, "Oh yes, everyone here is just wonderful."

"She was really too cheerful," Amanda says. "I suspected something was wrong."

Louise had always been sociable, not a loner by anybody's definition, so when they visited, Amanda and John were dismayed to find that she did not participate in any of the activities offered at the facility. She ate her meals alone and then went back to her room. Before long, she was confined to a wheelchair.

On one of Amanda and John's visits, Louise introduced one of the male assistants in such glowing terms that Amanda became suspicious. After examining Louise carefully, they thought they saw bruises, but she denied being mistreated.

John and Amanda drove the seven hours back to St. Louis in almost complete silence, both of them wondering the same things. *What's going on at the nursing home? Why has Mom deteriorated so rapidly? Could something be that wrong at a church-owned facility? How could they be sure?*

Amanda finally broke the silence. "John, I think your mother is being abused."

"I know," said John. "I do too."

Caregiver Dilemmas

Conscientious caregivers are always hesitant to entrust the care of their loved ones to others, but third-party care is sometimes a necessity. It is fair to say that most nursing home management teams have the best interests of their clients at heart and that most nurses and nursing aides are conscientious people. Yet it is impossible for every caregiving activity to be directly monitored. Caregivers must trust those to whom they commit the care of their loved ones. Distance complicates every aspect of caregiving, and none more so than ensuring the safety of the care receiver under the charge of a nursing facility or other caregiving agent. Here are some vexing questions that plague long-distance caregivers.

Decision Making

Joyce's husband, Eugene, had a stroke, and was to be discharged from the hospital to a nursing home for further rehabilitation. Joyce visited several nursing homes looking for one that would provide the aggressive therapy Eugene would need in order to make the best use of his weakened arm and leg. One nursing home showed her a room full of shiny exercise equipment. It looked good. She asked if they had a physical therapist on staff, but the director's answer was vague. Another nursing home was a plain little place with plastic flowers on the table in the lobby. It had no shiny equipment, but it did have a physical therapist; however, he came in only two days a week. *What should I do?* Joyce wondered.

Frustration

Betty's father, Luther, is six feet tall. He used to weigh 210 pounds but is now down to145 pounds, too little for someone his height. He has dementia and is a nursing home patient in Betty's hometown, Maryville, Tennessee, about three and a half hours from her present home in Lexington, Kentucky. She visits her father every few weeks and keeps bringing his weight-loss problem to the attention of the nursing home staff. They thank her very much for her interest and do nothing. With great effort, she has persuaded the home to give him extra feedings of Ensure, a high-nutrition drink. Thankfully, Luther has gained some weight, but Betty does not know how often he gets the Ensure because she cannot be there every day to monitor his progress. How can she get the staff to follow through on the care plan?

Minimizing

One day when Mildred was visiting her mother, Suzanna, in the nursing home, her mother's roommate called Mildred to her bedside. "Your mother has trouble breathing sometimes. If I tell the nurses, I will not be believed. Please check into it."

Mildred discovered it was true. Her mother was having breathing problems.

"What if I had not taken the lady seriously?" Mildred asks. "One of the many frustrations of aging," she observes, "is loss of credibility. It's difficult to get anyone to believe you know what you are talking about when you are old and a nursing home patient."

If your mother raises an issue with the staff, will she be taken seriously?

Mistakes

Human beings make mistakes. Being short handed and over-worked can cause medication errors by the nursing staff. If the patient cannot monitor his or her own drugs, serious mistakes are possible. The long-distance caregiver is at a severe disadvantage because there is no way to be present even every day, let alone every time medications are dispensed. How can long-distance caregivers know if their loved ones are receiving proper medication?

Improper Feeding

The nursing home reports that your mother won't eat. You wonder if she won't eat or if she cannot feed herself and the facility staff is stretched so thin that no one can spend enough time with her to be sure she gets enough to eat. Are her food trays being delivered and then picked up twenty minutes later, untouched, because she can no longer remember how to handle a fork? Living four hours away, you can't be present for even one meal a day. How can you be sure she will get enough to eat?

Guilt

One day Virginia came into her mom's nursing home room just in time to see an attendant slap her mother. She reported the incident to the nursing home director and to her mother's doctor. The attendant was reprimanded but not fired.

Virginia feels torn. Transferring to another nursing home would involve lots of maneuvering and paper work–a huge hassle–and probably result in an even longer trip than the one hour she must now drive to see her mother. Yet Virginia is uneasy about leaving her mother in the present facility. "Am I leaving her there for her benefit," she asks, "or because it makes my life easier?"

Evaluating Skilled Nursing Facilities

Nothing illustrates the essence of Christianity like caring for and protecting the helpless. Jesus depicted that perfectly in His story of the Good Samaritan (Luke 10:30–37). Was the Good Samaritan the original long-distance caregiver?

We all know the story as Jesus set if forth. A man was going from Jerusalem to Jericho when he fell victim to robbers who beat him and left him bleeding. A priest and a Levite both passed by their injured fellow Jew, doing nothing to help him. It was the despised Gentile, the Samaritan, who took pity on the man, bound up his wounds, set the man on the Samaritan's own donkey, brought the fellow to an inn, and paid the innkeeper in advance for the man's care, promising to pay any additional costs on his return trip.

After the Samaritan left the wounded man in the innkeeper's care, do you suppose he wondered about any of the questions that long-distance caregivers so often rehearse? What if the innkeeper didn't take care of the man? What if he mistreated the defenseless patient? What if he pocketed the money but refused to provide adequate care? Was it a mistake to leave the man and trust the innkeeper? What if . . .

We could manufacture what-if questions indefinitely.

Jesus' hearers probably identified with the fallen victim, for their roads were infested with robbers. Many of us can identify with the Samaritan, for we are often tasked with providing for the care of loved ones, ensuring that they receive care we cannot provide ourselves. Even though we have telephones, like the Samaritan, we cannot be present every minute as caregivers. Ultimately, we are thrown back on the same resource for dealing with those what-if questions as was the Samaritan: trust in God. We remember that part of the reason Christ came was "to shine on those living in darkness and in the shadow of death, to guide our feet into the path of peace" (Luke 1:79). We must trust God–and trust others–to care for our loved ones when we cannot. Often, that is the only solution, and it is a biblical one. After all, God *is* trustworthy.

Evaluate the Facility Carefully

While we trust God, ultimately, for our own well being and that of our loved ones, there are, however, some practical things that long-distance caregivers can do to ensure the safety and adequate care of their loved ones. Here are some things you can do to evaluate a nursing facility before placing your loved one in its care.

1. Most nursing homes will give prospective clients a guided tour. By all means, take their tour. They will show you the good points. Go back later, unannounced, and wander down all the units looking in more detail at items that may pertain to your loved one. For example, if your care receiver often becomes confused and is inclined to wander, be sure there is a security system at the facility.

2. Take note of the smell. If the place smells bad, it is a sign that incontinent patients are not being promptly attended to.

3. Observe the dining room at mealtime. See what the meals look like. Make sure they provide enough protein and variety.

4. Find out how long patients who are unable to feed themselves must wait before someone comes to feed them. Also look to see if there are patients who have trays of food in front of them but are unable to eat. Notice whether the tray is taken away with the food untouched.

5. Observe the manner in which patients are fed. Notice whether the pace is too fast for the patient or so slow that the food is cold before it is eaten. Make sure patients are not denied liquids. Notice whether the caregivers tell patients what they are being fed. For example, a caregiver might say, "Now here is a bite of mashed potatoes."

6. Observe the hallways. Passageways that are clogged with wheelchairs, medicine carts, and other obstructions will be a hazard in the event of an emergency evacuation.

7. Notice the length of time patients are left unattended in wheelchairs.

8. Listen to the tone of voice of the caregivers. They should be respectful when addressing patients.

9. Ask to see a copy of the last state inspection report. This report is inconclusive, because nursing homes are warned of inspections, but it will help to get a picture of the facility's quality. You have the right to see this report.

10. Ask what the staff of the nursing home would do if your care receiver becomes disturbed or agitated or starts yelling. A poor solution would be to put the patient in restraints or administer drugs as a first resort. A good first treatment would be to institute calming procedures, such as a short walk or a snack. Ask if the nursing home is a "non-restraint facility."

11. If there is a locked unit, find out if any staff member responds when a patient pounds on the door. If the nursing

home is set on following their routine in every situation, don't place your loved one there.

12. Ask about the institution's ratio of staff members to patients. This is set by law and varies from state to state. A typical number is one helper to every twenty-two patients in an assisted living facility. In a skilled nursing home, a typical ratio is one to ten, with one registered nurse for every thirty patients. Ask the facility whether their ratio is a goal only or if that number is consistently maintained.

13. Find out whether or not the nursing home accepts Medicaid. When care receivers outlive their personal financial resources, it is difficult to uproot them and move them to a new place.

Keep in Constant Contact

Finding a good facility will go a long way toward ensuring the proper care of a loved one. But it is best to maintain purposeful involvement with your care receiver, even after placing him or her in skilled nursing care. Here are some things you can do to ensure the ongoing proper care of your loved one.

1. Let management know if your loved one is a wanderer or claustrophobic.

2. Ask about and be prepared to discuss your loved one's treatment plan. Find out all you can about your care receiver's ailments. Ask the doctor or nurse, get information at the local library, or go to medical sites on the internet like www.mywebmd.com or the National Institutes of Health at www.nih.gov for reliable medical information intended for lay persons.

3. Make frequent trips to visit—the more often, the better. If you cannot visit often, call the nurses' station in your care

receiver's section frequently and ask for a report. Keep on top of things as best you can.

4. If you cannot visit frequently, try to arrange for a friend living nearby to make occasional visits and report to you.

5. Get acquainted with the nurses and aides. Get to know your care receiver's doctor's nurse as well. He or she can be invaluable in checking things out for you at the nursing home.

6. On your visits, be attentive but not demanding, or you may alienate the nursing staff. For example, if you demand that a busy nurse immediately replenish the ice in your mother's water pitcher, you may create difficulty for your care receiver. If your request is reasonable, take note of how difficult it is or how much time it takes to find a staff person to help you.

7. When you visit, look for bruises on the body of your loved one.

8. If your care receiver can use a telephone, have one installed if at all possible. Ask for a type of service that prevents unauthorized toll calls.

9. Ask questions of your care receiver. Listen closely for tone-of-voice clues.

10. If you note mental confusion and suspect that it is caused by medication, request that a doctor review the care receiver's medications and evaluate his or her response to them.

11. Make an effort to go with your care receiver to doctor appointments. If you cannot be there, try to be represented by a family member. Ask that person to take notes on what is said and done.

12. Be certain that the care receiver takes a list of current medications and dosages to doctor appointments. If prescriptions have no refills left, this should be pointed out.

13. Make a list of questions for the physician and take them with you to appointments. If it is impossible for you or a family member to visit the doctor and if the doctor has a policy of not taking or returning phone calls from patients or their families, a last resort would be to mail or e-mail the questions to the physician.

14. Follow up on test results. Ask the care receiver's doctor how he or she prefers to make results available to you—by fax or mailed to you in a self-addressed, stamped envelope.

15. Maintain a list of the care receiver's current physicians, including their names, addresses, and telephone numbers.

16. Request that you be notified of any major change in the care receiver's condition.

17. If you believe that your care receiver is being abused in a long-term medical facility, consult with your local law enforcement agency. Be aware that there are legal ways to install a hidden camera in your loved one's room, but making an audio tape of conversations without informing the persons involved is illegal unless you have obtained a search warrant. Carefully consider whether or not to inform the facility's administrators of your suspicions and actions. A good facility will be eager to root out any mistreatment. A poor one may be less cooperative.

Tender Mercies

Not long after Amanda and John Parker visited Louise in the assisted living unit of her Wichita nursing home, the home reported that Louise could no longer dress herself, kept falling, was unable to walk to the dining room, and had become incontinent. The facility's managers insisted that she be moved to the skilled nursing section of the home. In skilled care, Louise would have a roommate, something John and Amanda knew would be very hard on Louise. It would also be much more expensive. Faced with the choice of going into skilled care in Wichita or moving to St. Louis, nearer to her son and daughter-in-law, Louise chose to move to St. Louis. Amanda and John placed Louise in another church-related retirement community, this one only ten minutes from their home. Louise entered the assisted living section, and John or Amanda stopped by every day to see her.

After moving to St. Louis, Louise admitted that she had been abused in the Wichita home. The attendant had hit her occasionally because she did not obey him fast enough. She also reported that although she could walk, the staff of the previous home had compelled her to use a wheelchair because she could be transported faster that way.

"Nobody wanted to take time to walk with me to meals," Louise said. She was quiet a few minutes, then added in an embarrassed whisper, "You know why I wet my bed at night? It was because we had supper at 5:00 p.m. and then had to go to bed at 6:00 p.m. I would ring the bell, but nobody ever came to help me to the bathroom at night . . . I just couldn't wait until morning."

Amanda and John realized also that Louise had become withdrawn at the previous facility out of fear. At the new place, in the loving atmosphere created by a dedicated staff of nurses and aides, Louise blossomed. She took walks in the corridors, sat in the sunshine on the back porch, and chatted with new friends. On her birthday, Amanda and John gave a big party and invited everybody in the assisted living unit.

Louise lived only six weeks in her new location before dying suddenly of an aortic hemorrhage. But the time remains a happy memory for her son and daughter-in-law.

"I'm so glad Mom didn't die abused and alone," says Amanda. "We thank the Lord for His mercies."

Chapter Thirteen

Your Dog Has Fleas
Cherishing Family Memories

Distance Dilemma	Maintaining family memories as loved ones drift apart.
Caregiver Connection	*Seize the opportunity to record priceless family history.*

Claudia Haviland was married in an elegant evening ceremony, with tall tapers adorning the end of each pew. "I'm told that they needed every inch of height," says her daughter, Patricia Bradford-Burton, "because mother was always late."

From an affluent background, a graduate of Wellesley, an expert swimmer and diver, a writer of poetry, Claudia Haviland had been one of the most sought-after young women in Cambridge, Massachusetts, in the 1920s. Claudia had rejected thirteen offers of marriage before accepting the hand of James Bradford. "He was English," says Patricia. "He was very bright, very fun, just the sort of person mother would fall for." He was also a "Cunarder," having taken to sea on a sailing vessel at the age of sixteen. Armed with lots of books, the gift of an aunt, he read eagerly, educating himself aboard ship. He became an officer on various ships of the Cunard line and was promoted to captain just before he died of throat cancer at the age of forty-two, leaving Claudia with three young children.

"Mother never remarried," Patricia says. "I don't think she ever met anyone else who could keep up with her—that woman was something else."

Claudia, who had lived and worked in New York City before her marriage, came back to the United States after her husband's death. She settled the family in Rye, New York, and became a copy editor for *Time* magazine, a job that demanded breadth of knowledge, exacting standards of accuracy, and superb editorial skill. Patricia remembers her mother being at home most evenings and the family eating dinner together regularly.

Decades passed. Claudia retired to Florida and began yet another phase of her storied life, settling in Sarasota, famous as the winter home of the Ringling Bros. Circus. "I didn't really know much about Mom's life in Florida," Patricia says now. "It was wonderful to be able to escape the winter at Mom's house down there, but for years, that's all it was—a pleasant break."

Claudia's life in Florida was nothing if not active. She began to lose her hearing, but learned to lip-read very well and continued to enjoy attending lectures. She took art history courses at the local university. She was active with the Audubon Society, and got into the local politics of saving bird sanctuaries. She was a docent at the Ringling Museum. Claudia, at age eighty-four, sailed around the world on the steamship *Queen Elizabeth 2* and had a knee replaced successfully the next year.

But, inevitably, Claudia's health began to deteriorate. As her deafness became complete, Claudia depended on her little dog,

Goldie, to alert her when someone was at the door. "The fact that Goldie carried fleas into the house did not trouble Mom," says Patricia. "For some reason the fleas did not bite her." One January when Patricia went to Sarasota, she discovered that the palm rats that normally live outside in the palm trees had taken up residence in her mother's attic and had eaten a hole in the ceiling. "Palm rats have very large droppings," she added dryly. But that didn't bother Claudia, who continued to live her independent, capricious life.

Patricia's trips to Sarasota became more frequent and more focused on caring for her aging mother. Rather than relaxing, reading, or enjoying the beach, Patricia's time was taken with managing household affairs, persuading Claudia to hire the help she refused to believe was needed, and scheduling medical treatments—the usual duties of long-distance caregiving.

Yet as Claudia's health continued to decline, Patricia began to worry. "Not so much about losing Mom," Patricia says. "I knew she wouldn't live forever. I worried about losing her presence in my life. She had traveled so much and seen so much and experienced so much—what would life be like when she was gone?"

Paying Attention to Wisdom

The Bible applauds listening to our elders. "Listen to your father, who gave you life, and do not despise your mother when she is old," says Solomon (Prov. 23:22). Moses teaches respect for the aged in the same breath with revering God. He quotes God's words to him: "Rise in the presence of the aged, show respect for the elderly and revere your God. I am the Lord" (Lev. 19:32).

Patricia says that even at the height of her hectic trips to Sarasota, she made occasions to sit down with her mother and talk about "the old days." She asked her mother to identify the people in family photos and quizzed her about life in the first half of the century. With tape recorder running, she interviewed her mother to fill in the gaps in the Haviland-Bradford family history.

The exercise paid rich dividends.

Preserving Family Identity

Patricia talked with her mother about her childhood in Massachusetts and her life in England as a young married woman. "When you got Mom started, you couldn't stop her," Patricia says. Long, tape-recorded conversations revealed a rich family history, a deposit Patricia now guards for her own children. If not for those interviews, many details of their heritage would have been lost. Patricia's children would have had no sense of their ancestors or their past. But now, as Patricia puts it, "They'll know who they are."

Seeing Parents as People

Yet Patricia sees a deeper reason to interview older persons, beyond gaining information. "It makes them feel like people when you listen to them," she says. "It's not enough to care for their physical needs; it's important to make them feel that their lives have had value."

Patricia quotes C. S. Lewis' book, *Out of the Silent Planet*:

But it takes [a man's] whole life. When he is young he has to look for his mate; and then he has to court her; then he begets young; then he rears them; then he remembers all this, and boils it inside him and makes it into poems and wisdom.

She comments, "I think part of our ministry to older people is to value them enough to listen to their poems and wisdom. She is not just 'your mother.' She is a person whom you can get to know."

Forging a Family Bond

Lynn and Jerry, who spent nearly ten years shuttling between their home in Springfield, Massachusetts, to the home of Jerry's mother, Lillian Schneider, in Revere, also took the time to collect an oral history of their family. And they gained something more—an oral history of the twentieth century.

"I would say, 'Mom, tell us a new story,'" says Jerry. "And she would tell us more details about her flight from Germany with my father just prior to World War II." Both Jewish, they had escaped the Nazi regime by fleeing to Paris, then England. "She told us about living in England during the war, and about moving to the United States, where my father continued his work as a physicist," Jerry says.

"We felt enriched by the time spent talking with her," Lynn adds. "She gave something valuable to us."

On one of Jerry's visits to her home, Lillian, realizing the difficulty her son faced in commuting over an hour to be with her, called Lynn to say that she regretted taking Jerry away from her.

"But Mom," Lynn protested, "you already gave him to me—when we were married."

"Yes," she replied, "but you never took him," meaning that over the nearly four decades of their marriage, Lynn had never attempted to alienate her husband from his mother.

When Lillian died in Jerry's arms the following day, her comment from the previous evening became a loving summary of their shared relationship.

Sunrise, Sunset

Long-distance caregiving became a surreal experience for Patricia Bradford-Burton as her mother's life, always eccentric, descended into chaos. Claudia cooked only occasionally, paid bills rarely, and cleaned house never. "I thought the place had become a health hazard," Patricia reports. "Mom thought everything was fine."

One November, swamped with the Christmas rush at her family business, Patricia hired a woman named Anna, sight unseen, to live in the apartment over her mother's garage, cook dinner two or three times a week, clean house some, and check on Claudia each day. Patricia talked with Anna on the telephone only once, but she came well recommended. Her pastor had said that Anna was "a good person."

Almost immediately Patricia began to get calls from the neighbors complaining about the new housekeeper. As it turned out, Anna weighed more than three hundred pounds and was in the habit of washing out her enormous bloomers each day and hanging them on a clothesline strung across the neighbor's view of Sarasota bay.

Patricia, buried under a Massachusetts snowstorm, called Anna and asked her to please move the clothesline. One week later Patricia received a report that water was pouring through the garage ceiling. From Massachusetts, she called a plumber in Sarasota, who discovered that the rotund housekeeper's weight had cracked the toilet. Next, Claudia complained that her grocery bill had risen dramatically after Anna arrived. Then Anna complained that Claudia had been rude to her.

"It was like dealing with spatting children, but from a distance of fourteen hundred miles," Patricia recalls.

For better or worse, the Sarasota circus was short lived. After her mother died, Patricia's life returned to normal. Gone are the long journeys to Florida, the palm rats, and the corpulent housekeeper. Even little Goldie and her fleas are gone.

What remains is the memory of Claudia's unique identity—her strengths and weaknesses, her wisdom and whimsy, her legacy to her grandchildren. Amid the disarray and turmoil of caregiving, Patricia created an opportunity for her mother to share her wisdom as a debutante, global traveler, young widow, single mother, professional editor, and woman of the world. Patricia cherishes that wisdom, and will pass it on to her own children. Ask her about her mother sometime, and Patricia will gladly tell you: "That woman was something else."

Afterword

Several themes emerged through the dozens of interviews with long-distance caregivers who share their stories in this book. These persons, unknown to each other, repeated the same issues over and over in what became a kind of caregiving litany. Most of those statements are made clearly in the chapters of this book; I summarize them here because of their extreme importance. Some of these lessons reflect tender compassion for aging parents. Others are blunt warnings. All are the unvarnished opinions of persons who have been there. They are given in the approximate order of the frequency with which they were mentioned by caregivers.

Let Changes Be the Care Receivers' Decision

Be sure that any change made in the care receivers' lifestyle is for their good and not for the convenience of the caregiver. Care receivers, whether aging parents or others, should be included in the conversations regarding such plans. When the care receivers must move, perhaps from the house where they have lived for decades into a smaller, safer, more manageable space, make every effort to help them reach that conclusion on their own.

At the same time, it is important to develop a plan before you speak. If it is clear that a change must be made, it is best to present that need to the caregiver with a well-thought arrangement in mind. But be flexible. A compromise may have to be made.

Don't Sweat the Small Stuff

It is more important to maintain friendship with your siblings and parents than always to get your way on decisions affecting your care receivers. Do not rupture an irreplaceable family bond over something that you will later discover has small value. Remember, after parents are gone, siblings will remain. It is wise to keep their friendship.

When in Doubt, Go

Do not apologize because you had no specific reason for going to visit your parents or other care receivers. Visiting them is something that you do to benefit yourself as well as them. It is not wrong to make a trip for no reason other than your own peace of mind. Go for your own satisfaction without guilt or apology.

Mind Your Own Business

Resist the temptation to rearrange your parents' furniture, change their household routines, clean out their refrigerator, or engage in other busybodyish activities, no matter how noble your motives may be or how awkward their habits may appear.

Listen Sympathetically

If you are a caregiver who is only occasionally present and someone else has responsibility for primary care, don't offer advice to the primary caregiver unless specifically asked to do so. Instead, be attentive when the primary caregiver calls or e-mails.

Be a sympathetic, patient, listening ear, a soft shoulder to cry on. Let the primary caregiver unload his or her emotions on you.

Don't Worry about What Others Think

Do not be disturbed if outsiders think your arrangements for your parents are strange and volunteer lots of "good advice." Outsiders almost never know all the facts and seldom understand the dynamics of someone else's family. Thank them pleasantly for their ideas, and let it go at that.

When a decision is needed, make it. Go on, decide. Gather what information you can, pray about it, and make a choice. Most of the time, it will be right. If you choose correctly 75 percent of the time, you are about average. Don't beat yourself up later when a decision made in good faith turns out to be wrong.

Set Boundaries

If manipulation by a care receiver has been a problem in the past, set boundaries. That is, create emotional distance between yourself and the care receiver. By doing this, you avoid feeling undeserved guilt or anger. As a long-distance caregiver, the geographic distance may enable you to exercise a more positive influence on the management of your care receiver's treatment than if you were closer emotionally and physically.

However, in setting necessary boundaries, be certain that you do not swing to the extreme of becoming so aloof that the care receiver is afraid to approach you with a genuine problem.

Cherish the Days

Difficult as they now seem, these days will not last indefinitely. Amid the fatigue, frustration, and anxiety that accompany any caregiving experience, recognize the precious trust that God has given you—the care of another human being. Seek God's wisdom and strength; He will freely give them. And cherish these days while they last.

Glossary of Caregiving Terms

Advance Directive. A document that states the care receiver's choices about medical care, or names someone to make medical choices if the care receiver is unable to speak for him or herself. It is signed in advance of need so the family and doctors know how to proceed regarding medical treatment. Examples of advance directives include living wills, healthcare surrogate designations, durable powers of attorney, and living will directives.

Assisted Living. Sometimes called "personal care or "custodial care." A level of care given when the care receiver needs assistance with activities of daily living such as bathing, dressing, eating, and other routine activities. In a typical institutional setting, each assisted living resident has one room and a bath, often furnished with furniture from his or her old home. Attendants, who are usually persons without medical training, assist residents as needed. Assisted living may be provided in many settings, including nursing homes, adult day care centers, as one level of care in a retirement community, or in the care receiver's home.

Continuing Care Retirement Community. A for-profit or a non-profit community, often church related, which provides living quarters at three levels. These are fully independent living in apartments or free-standing duplexes or quadraplexes, often called cottages, patio homes, manors, or some similar designation;

assisted living rooms as described above; and a skilled nursing home service as described below. Typically there is a minimum age requirement, often sixty-five years. Many financial arrangements exist. A common plan is payment of a large upfront entrance fee, plus a monthly fee. In the assisted living and skilled nursing home levels of care, all meals, housekeeping, and laundry are provided. In the independent living level, one meal a day served in a common dining room is often included in the fee. In other communities, meals are optional and billed on an as-used basis. Housekeeping services may or may not be included. Laundry is usually not included, but apartments may be equipped with washers and dryers.

Custodial Care. See *Assisted Living.*

Durable Power of Attorney. See *Power of Attorney.*

Guardian. A person appointed by a court who is entrusted with the custody and control of someone who cannot act for him or herself. Those for whom guardians are appointed may be a child, a mentally ill person, a missing person, or one who is incompetent for any reason. A guardian is appointed only after extensive investigation by the court. A guardianship is regarded as a trust relation of a most sacred character, since the guardian is acting to represent and protect a person who cannot act for him or herself.

Healthcare Surrogates. A person the care receiver appoints in a written document to make medical decisions if he or she is unable to communicate.

Intermediate Nursing Care. A level of care for stable conditions that require daily, but not 24-hour nursing supervision. Such care is ordered by a physician and supervised by registered nurses. It is less specialized than skilled nursing care, and is often needed for a long period of time.

Living Will Directives. A document including any or all of the following: directions stating whether the care receiver does or does not wish life-prolonging treatment and/or food and water be provided artificially, that all or any part of the body be donated, and the name of the person or persons who are to act as surrogates, or decision makers.

Personal Care. See *Assisted Living.*

Power of Attorney. A document in which the care receiver gives another person the authority to perform certain acts on behalf of him or herself. The person named is called the attorney-in-fact. A durable power of attorney gives unlimited powers, and a limited power of attorney specifies only certain things that the holder of it can do. A durable power of attorney is a very powerful instrument. The person who holds it can sell the care receiver's house or car, and even empty out his or her bank account, with or without consent. A bank or other financial institution can be appointed to take an individual's power of attorney. That person or institution may or may not be empowered to make medical decisions for the care receiver, depending on how the document is worded. The power of attorney ends with the death of the maker. Sometimes abbreviated POA.

Retirement Community. See Continuing Care Retirement Community.

Skilled Nursing Care. Care for medical conditions that require skilled medical personnel, such as registered nurses or professional therapists. Such care is available twenty-four hours a day, is ordered by a physician, and involves a treatment plan. Skilled care may be provided in a nursing home or in a person's home with help from visiting nurses.

Trust. Created when property is transferred from the care receiver to another person or a banking corporation (the trustee) for the purpose of managing the property and its income for the benefit of a person or organization (the beneficiary). A trustee may assume many of the burdens of financial management.

Care Receiver's Information Packet

aregivers, whether long distance or close at hand, should keep the following information about the care receiver all together in one packet, readily available for use in an emergency. If the care receiver has a lawyer, copies of this information should be kept also in the lawyer's office.

Vital History

Full name, birth date, address, name and contact information for the person holding power of attorney, name and contact information for next of kin.

Family Information

Names and contact information for the care receiver's parents, children, siblings, or other family members and friends who should be notified in the event of the care receiver's serious illness or death. It may be helpful to name those who should *not* be notified as well.

Medical History

Current health problems; current medications, including the drug name, dosage, and frequency; known allergies; medicines to which the care receiver has shown an adverse reaction; surgical history.

Medical Information

Name, telephone number, and address for the care receiver's primary physician and any others from whom he or she is receiving care; pharmacy name and phone number; hospital preference.

Insurance Information

Copies (not originals) of the care receiver's Medicare card, secondary insurance card, and pharmacy coverage card; company name, policy number, and contact information for any life insurance policies on the care receiver; company name, policy number, and contact information for long-term care insurance provider, if any. Include a note telling where the original copies of insurance documents are kept.

Legal Information

Copies (not originals) of the care receiver's will, living will, power of attorney, and health care power of attorney; names and contact information for the person or persons holding the care receiver's power of attorney, health care power of attorney; contact information for the executor of the care receiver's will; a note telling the location of the original documents named in this section, the location of any safe deposit boxes held by the care receiver, and the location of the keys to any such safe deposit boxes; a valid Do Not Resuscitate (DNR) form, if desired by the care receiver. (Some states require a special form and will not recognize a living will as a DNR document.)

Business Information

Names, addresses, and telephone numbers of the care receiver's bank, broker, lawyer, accountant, or tax preparer, and employer or former employer under whom the care receiver might be insured or hold retirement accounts; names and contact information for business associates.

Funeral Information

Funeral preferences, if they have been stated by the care receiver; funeral home preference with contact information and details of any pre-arrangements that have been made; cemetery preference with contact information and details of any pre-arrangements; list of potential pallbearers; church or clergy preference with contact information. If cremation is chosen, specify instructions for the disposition of the ashes.

Ten Warning Signs of Caregiver Stress

From the Alzheimer's Association

1. *Denial* about the disease and its effects on the person who's been diagnosed. "I know Mom's going to get better."
2. *Anger* at the person with Alzheimer's or others: that no effective treatments or cures currently exist, and that people don't understand what's going on. "If he asks me that question one more time, I'll scream."
3. *Social withdrawal* from friends and activities that once brought pleasure. "I don't care about getting together with the neighbors anymore."
4. *Anxiety* about facing another day and what the future holds. "What happens when he needs more care than I can provide?"
5. *Depression* begins to break your spirit and affects your ability to cope. "I don't care anymore."
6. *Exhaustion* makes it nearly impossible to complete necessary daily tasks. "I'm too tired for this."
7. *Sleeplessness* caused by a never-ending list of concerns. "What if she wanders out of the house or falls and hurts herself?"

8. *Irritability* leads to moodiness and triggers negative responses and reactions. "Leave me alone!"

9. *Lack of concentration* makes it difficult to perform familiar tasks. "I was so busy, I forgot we had an appointment."

10. *Health problems* begin to take their toll, both mentally and physically. "I can't remember the last time I felt good."